'This very important book showcases accurately a giant stride this project achieved in moving people living with dementia from participants to leaders in the world of dementia research. As someone fortunate to have been closely involved in one project, and knowing the pioneers and the book's authors well, I cannot commend this game-changing initiative highly enough. For the first time, people living with dementia were placed at the centre with their needs, wishes, aspirations, talent and commitment encouraged and supported to lead answering questions we all are asking and can benefit from answering – that is genuine research. Let us all hope the baton it is handing over will be taken further.'

– Keith Oliver, author of *Dear Alzheimer's:*
A Diary of Living with Dementia

'People living with dementia know better than anyone what will help to improve their experience. This ground-breaking and heart-warming project shows the potential of putting people with dementia "in the driving seat" of enquiry. It challenges researchers and research funders to rethink involvement and work in genuine partnership.'

– Linda Clare, Professor of Clinical
Psychology of Ageing and Dementia University of Exeter

'This book is both a challenge to move beyond co-production in research and a guide to how we can achieve it. The questions posed and lessons shared apply not just to research but to how we work together with people with dementia in all aspects of our work.'

– Colin Capper, Associate Director of Evidence
and Involvement, Alzheimer's Society

T0385332

'This inspirational book marks the emergence of a new research culture for dementia studies. It is essential reading for the research community, policymakers and students of health and social care.'

– Richard Ward, Senior Lecturer in Dementia Studies,
University of Stirling

'An essential read for researchers and academics challenging the myths and misconceptions about the ability of people with dementia to actively participate in research. The Dementia Enquirers Gold Standards are excellent and should be used to guide *all* dementia research.'

– Dr Hilda Hayo, Chief Admiral Nurse and
CEO Dementia UK

'This account of the Dementia Enquirers Project has inspired me, and given me excellent resources, to go further in working together with people living with dementia in my own research career.'

– Jan Oyebode, Professor of Dementia Care,
University of Bradford

People with Dementia at the Heart of Research

People with Dementia at the Heart of Research

Co-Producing Research through
The Dementia Enquirers Model

Rachael Litherland
and **Philly Hare**

Foreword by Dr David Crepaz-Keay

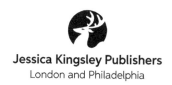

Jessica Kingsley Publishers
London and Philadelphia

First published in Great Britain in 2024 by Jessica Kingsley Publishers
An imprint of John Murray Press

I

Copyright © Rachael Litherland and Philly Hare 2024

Foreword copyright © David Crepaz-Keay 2024

The right of Rachael Litherland and Philly Hare to be identified as
the Author of the Work has been asserted by them in accordance
with the Copyright, Designs and Patents Act 1988.

Front cover image source: AdobeStock.

A CIP catalogue record for this title is available from the
British Library and the Library of Congress

ISBN 978 1 78775 702 8
eISBN 978 1 78775 703 5

Printed and bound by CPI Group (UK) Ltd, Croydon, CR0 4YY

Jessica Kingsley Publishers' policy is to use papers that are natural,
renewable and recyclable products and made from wood grown in
sustainable forests. The logging and manufacturing processes are expected
to conform to the environmental regulations of the country of origin.

Jessica Kingsley Publishers
Carmelite House
50 Victoria Embankment
London EC4Y 0DZ

www.jkp.com

John Murray Press
Part of Hodder & Stoughton Ltd
An Hachette Company

Contents

Foreword

It is a great pleasure and privilege for me to write the foreword for this remarkable book, which highlights the ground-breaking work of a group of people living with dementia who have become knowledge creators. This book tells a unique and inspiring story of how they harnessed the experience of living with dementia, and the stigma, discrimination and negative stereotypes that so often accompany it.

As someone who has walked this path in the mental health world, I have witnessed the transformative effect of research on both individuals and society. However, this book takes this impact to new and exciting places, by demonstrating how people living with dementia can not only contribute to research, but also become respected academics in their own right. By promoting the voice of people living with dementia as knowledge builders, this book calls for a more inclusive approach to research, and reminds us of the power of collaboration across disciplines and stakeholders.

In recent years, there has been a growing recognition of the importance in research of involving people with lived experience. This book advances this thinking by demonstrating the practical value of including people living with dementia as academic researchers. The book spans the full range of academic fields, showcasing an array of research methods and topics conducted by people living with dementia, including qualitative, quantitative and arts-based methods.

Readers will learn many lessons from this book and everyone will have their favourites. For me there are a couple that have made a lasting impression. The first is the way the Enquirers moved from seeing academic ethics as a block to involvement in research, to writing an influential guide to how ethics should be done properly. The second is challenging my own prejudice (and that of most people I know) that dementia is all about memory loss. When people living with dementia really control the research agenda, then we discover the full range of meaningful research questions (no more spoilers, read the book and learn!).

I know that, if I spend some of my life living with dementia, then that experience will be much better as a result of reading this book, and, more particularly, as a result of the remarkable work of the Pioneers, Enquirers and the authors of this book who helped to make it happen.

I cannot recommend this book highly enough, and I hope that it will be widely read and discussed by those who fund research, the academic community, policymakers and the general public. It is a truly ground-breaking contribution to our understanding of dementia, research and the human spirit.

Dr David Crepaz-Keay
March 2023

Acknowledgements

We'd like to thank the National Lottery Community Fund for giving us this amazing and ground-breaking opportunity – we hope we've done them proud; and also the many academics, and others, who have supported us with huge enthusiasm and a lot of practical guidance. They have helped us to navigate the labyrinthine world of research (Wendy Mitchell, Pioneer).

The Pioneers

Peter Berry

Daithi Cee

Teresa (Dory) Davies

Irene Donaldson

Carol Fordyce

Howard Gordon

Agnes Houston MBE

Steve Kennedy

Rev. Mhari McLintock

Dr Wendy Mitchell

Masood (Maq) Qureshi

George Rook

Tracey Shorthouse

Programme advisors

Dr Rosie Ashworth (Tayside NHS)

Professor Dawn Brooker MBE (Worcester University)

Dr David Crepaz-Keay (Mental Health Foundation)

Dr Lucy Series (Cardiff University)

Professor Tom Shakespeare (London School of Hygiene and Tropical Medicine)

Experts involved in the development of the Dementia Enquirers Gold Standards for Ethical Research

Dr Laura Booi (Newcastle University)

Susan Harrison (former Vice-Chair, Social Care Research Ethics Committee)

Dr Jody Mellor (Disability Research on Independent Living and Learning Programme Officer, Disability Wales)

Dr Caroline Norrie (King's College London)

Bridget Penhale (University of East Anglia)

Dr Martin Stevens (King's College London)

Dr Elizabeth Tilley (the Open University)

Professor Val Williams (retired, University of Bristol)

Toby Williamson (consultant)

Professor Tracey Williamson (University of Worcester)

And finally, of course, our congratulations to the 21 Dementia Engagement and Empowerment Project (DEEP) groups which have pioneered the 'driving seat' approach by leading their own research projects.

CHAPTER 1

The Background to Dementia Enquirers

It's our opportunity to amaze people with what we can do. It's about coming together on our terms. (Martin)

Chapter summary

Research is the creation of new knowledge – or the use of existing knowledge in a new and creative way – to generate new ideas and understanding. Dementia Enquirers is an ambitious and novel programme of work which has tested out what it means for people with dementia to be those 'knowledge creators'. In this chapter, we describe the rationale of the programme, including the experiences of people with dementia of being involved in research. We look at alternative research approaches from disability studies and user-led research. We also describe some of the foundations for people with dementia being 'in the driving seat' of research.

Note: Throughout the book the word 'we' is used to mean the group that shaped the programme throughout. This included the Pioneers (people living with dementia), Innovations in Dementia staff and our advisors/allies. Although the book has technically been authored by Innovations in Dementia staff, the content has been co-produced by all those involved.

Involving people with dementia in research

It is not that long ago that even the idea of including people with dementia as research participants was up for debate. At the turn of the century, researchers were only just beginning to try out ways of asking the views of people with dementia in research settings.

Conversations around these approaches included ethical and practical considerations such as:

- gaining informed consent
- the risks associated with involvement
- the validity of responses from people with dementia.

A number of pioneering researchers worked hard to bring the voices of people with dementia into research, testing out and learning about the best ways to do this (Wilkinson, 2001). They challenged not only the research system but also the prevailing stigmatizing narratives about people with dementia. It was people with dementia who showed them the way, by sharing their experiences and having their perspectives included in research.

Fast forward to 2023. The experiences of people with dementia are reflected in a range of research studies, with researchers needing to be explicit about the ethical approaches they adopt to make this a good and safe experience. Additionally, there is a much higher expectation, particularly from research funders, that people with dementia should not just be the subjects of research, but should also have a *stake in* research – a say in what it is and how it is carried out.

Dementia Enquirers is an innovative programme that has created knowledge, principles and standards around co-research with people with dementia, moving beyond 'patient and public involvement and engagement' and co-production, to a model where people with dementia are in the driving seat of research. We will begin by describing some of the reasons why we developed the Dementia Enquirers programme.

'Patient and public involvement and engagement'

Much dementia research is still dominated by the medical model, which regards disability as an impairment, as a deviation from 'normal' health status. The focus is on neurodegeneration and brain pathology, and the central message is that the resulting dementias need to be treated, cured, fixed or at least rehabilitated.

While it used to be the case that family members were asked to act as proxies for people with dementia, the latter are increasingly being included in research studies and their own views and experiences sought. Many people with dementia commit to research participation following their diagnosis, with initiatives such as Join Dementia Research matching them up to research opportunities. People often say how enjoyable they find research participation and how they want to give something back, while hopefully improving things for future generations of people with dementia. Martin captures this in his quote which opens this chapter.

However, most large research and academic funding bodies do now make 'patient and public involvement and engagement' (PPIE) a condition of giving out their money. PPIE means members of the public informing and shaping research. It is different from taking part in research as a participant.

PPIE can (and should) happen even before the research starts, with academic researchers encouraged to talk with people to find out the issues that are most important to them. However, in our experience this doesn't happen very often!

PPIE makes research better. Researchers can connect with people with dementia to get advice on their research methods and project materials, and to discuss findings, recommendations and dissemination. A PPIE group of people with dementia that meets regularly with researchers can really change the way the research unfolds. For academics, their research is more efficient, effective and impactful. PPIE can help them communicate their findings more effectively, and generally make research more accessible to all.

High-quality PPIE is now usually an expectation of funders. For example, the National Institute for Health and Care Research (NIHR) states that public involvement is at the centre of its research and recommends there to be a named person with appropriate skills and experience who is responsible for leading PPIE within a research project. The NIHR (2021) sets out its own reasons why PPIE is important:

- *Democratic principles:* people who are affected by research have a right to have a say in it. It's part of citizenship, public accountability and transparency. It can also help to empower people by providing the opportunity to influence research that is relevant to them.

- *Providing a different perspective:* personal knowledge and experience bring a different perspective to the research. People are not just their health condition – they bring other life experiences as well.
- *Improving the quality of the research:* involving 'patients and the public' helps ensure that research focuses on outcomes that are important to people.
- *Making the research more relevant:* this occurs by identifying a wider set of research topics than would have been generated by just academics, ensuring that research is focused on both what matters to people and helping to shape and clarify the research.
- *Interests of research funders and research organizations:* several funding bodies, as well as research ethics committees (RECs), ask grant applicants about their plans for PPIE. There are high expectations that PPIE is a consideration of funding applications (or there is a good reason why this is not the case).
- *Ethics:* RECs will often ask about plans for PPIE. It may even be part of their assessment process. They too have high expectations that it is considered and planned, as it can help ensure that research is ethical, relevant and acceptable from a public perspective.

We should mention that people with dementia have said they don't really like the term 'PPIE'. First, it is an acronym, and people rarely know what it stands for. Second, it refers to patients and the public. People with dementia tend not to identify as 'patients' unless they are in a healthcare situation.

Emancipatory research

In the wider disability field, it is increasingly the case that people who use services, rather than professionals, are not just *involved in*, but *have control over*, the research process. They plan and undertake research and interpret the findings.

Emancipatory research, as it is known, sets out to empower the people who are usually the subjects of research. In 1992, disability rights activist Mike Oliver coined the phrase 'emancipatory disability research' to refer to a radical new approach to researching disability connected to the social model of disability.

According to Barnes (2001), the emancipatory research agenda warrants the 'transformation of the material and social relations of research production' – that is, the way that research is delivered, the way that research questions are formulated and the way that research is funded. Disabled people and disability organizations rather than professionals and academic researchers should have control of research agendas. Emancipatory research should be judged by its ability to empower disabled people through the research process.

We can see principles from emancipatory research ideas in practice in several different projects. For example, the Mental Health Foundation's 'Strategies for Living' project launched in 1997. Its aim was to document and disseminate people's strategies for living with mental distress in all its forms (Faulkner & Layzell, 2000). A core part of the project was to support people with mental health issues to carry out their own small-scale research.

In 2019, Tuffrey-Wijne and colleagues at Kingston and St George's University ran a training course for people with mild to moderate learning disabilities. They called it 'Learning How to do Research'. The course focused on understanding the research process and gaining practical skills in collecting, analysing and presenting data. Training methods were experimental, with an emphasis on interactive, hands-on learning. Students developed their own research questions, gathered data and presented their findings. Six months after completing the course, the graduates reported that they had better knowledge of research and had increased their skills. The students had greater self-esteem. Several of the students went on to take up new work opportunities.

DRILL[1] (Disability Research on Independent Living and Learning) was a UK-wide programme of research and pilot projects run between 2015 and 2020 by, for and about disabled people. This initiative promoted co-production and collaboration between disabled people and their organizations, academia, research bodies and policymakers. Disabled people were empowered to have direct influence on policies, legislation and services. The aim of the project was to create a body of work that explored some of the issues affecting disabled people and how they

---

1   www.drilluk.org.uk

might be resolved. Thirty-two projects were funded to find solutions for how disabled people can live as full citizens and take part socially, economically and politically. Over 300 disabled people were leaders of DRILL projects, through which they found new jobs, learned new skills, increased their confidence and felt as if they mattered.

There are also quite a few examples of older people leading research. In a 2006 study, 22 older people were the core interviewers on a project called Housing Decisions in Old Age. They trained over a two-term research methods course and carried out 189 in-depth interviews (Clough et al., 2006). Buffel and James (2019) worked with older people as co-researchers on a project to develop age-friendly communities. The project involved 18 older people who took a leading role in all phases of the study. The co-researchers completed 68 interviews with residents aged 60 and over who were experiencing social isolation within their neighbourhood. This led to important findings about how the community could be made more age-friendly.

A systematic review of older people as co-researchers (James & Buffel, 2022) suggested that research involvement:

- improves understanding of the issues facing older people
- offers more improved and responsive policy, practice and service design
- provides opportunities for people to develop new skills
- gives voice to marginalized groups of older people.

Much has been written about emancipatory research, and there has been plenty of criticism, particularly of its most purist approach. Where more experiential research is undertaken, it is still considered by many to be a realistic aim for researchers to be impartial – to operate in the most unbiased and value-free way as possible. But emancipatory research assumes that there are multiple realities and that research is not built only by an elite or dominant researcher. It questions the theoretical underpinnings of knowledge and methods, inquires beyond prevailing assumptions and understandings, and acknowledges the role of power in health and research.

All this has been changing the nature of research and knowledge, and what we recognize as 'evidence'. It has highlighted that we have often been asking the wrong questions – or looking through the wrong lens!

Emancipatory research, as a research perspective, provides a foundation of theory that can support people with dementia to take more control of research, and to be creators of research themselves. We will explore these shifts of power and control in dementia research, first by examining the approach of co-production.

Co-production

It is increasingly the case in the 'disability field' that people who use services, rather than professionals, have control over the research process (Staley, 2009). It is far from unusual now that disabled and/or older people plan and undertake research, and interpret the findings. But in the 'dementia world' progress has been much slower. And although PPIE is a big step forward, people with dementia say that their experience of it is varied.

It can make them question whether they are actually just being used in a tokenistic way to meet the requirements of funders, and to 'tick the box' for inclusion. Others are grateful for the inclusion, so are maybe blind to the inappropriate use of their time. However, sometimes it is a real joy.

In recent times, there have been opportunities for people with dementia to be more involved in research as co-investigators and co-producers. Co-production means different things to different people and is quite hard to define. But essentially it is about:

- getting involved as equals
- being recognized for the experience you bring
- making something happen together.

It is not just about participating in other people's work or ideas but helping to shape things from the beginning. It is about sharing power and control.

In co-production, researchers, practitioners and the public work together, bringing their different expertise to the pot. The New Economics Foundation (2008, p.6) describes co-production as:

Where professionals and citizens share power to design, plan, assess and deliver support together. It recognizes that *everyone has a vital contribution to make* [emphasis added] in order to improve quality of life for people and communities.

The NIHR's (2021) description of the key principles of co-production can be summarized as:

- Sharing of power: the research is jointly owned and people work together to achieve a joint understanding.
- Including all perspectives and skills: the research team must include all those who can make a contribution.
- Respecting and valuing the knowledge of all those working together on the research: everyone is of equal importance.
- Reciprocity: everybody benefits from working together.
- Building and maintaining relationships: there is an emphasis on relationships being key to sharing power. There needs to be joint understanding and consensus, and clarity of roles and responsibilities. It is also important to value people and unlock their potential.

Examples of co-production include IDEAL (Improving the Experience of Dementia and Enhancing Active Life, University of Exeter), the Neighbourhoods and Dementia Project (University of Manchester) and the Angela Project. In the IDEAL research programme, a PPIE group called ALWAYs (Action on Living Well: Asking You) plays a key role in the study. They advise on various aspects of the research based on their first-hand experiences, skills and expertise, influencing the research and how the findings are shared. Research funders have become increasingly supportive of co-production, and often perceive it as a natural next step to PPIE – if it is done well.

It feels as if the power is shifting. The Pioneers have said that these opportunities can be very enjoyable and satisfying, making them feel valued:

> After all, they give us a chance to work in a direct way with academic researchers, influencing and shaping research…if allowed.

Some case studies of co-production

In January 2021, the UK was in a lockdown due to Covid-19 restrictions. At the same time, a team of people with dementia began work to create a new resource to help newly diagnosed people with dementia identify their own goals and strategies. The idea for this resource came out of some research about cognitive rehabilitation (GREAT Cognitive Rehabilitation, University of Exeter[2]). Cognitive rehabilitation is a type of therapy that can make managing everyday activities easier for people in the earlier stages of dementia. It is often delivered via sessions with a therapist and can help people to identify and achieve, in a step-by-step way, the goals that are important to them.

With two researchers and Rachael Litherland from Innovations in Dementia, nine people with dementia worked together over eight months to talk, learn, share, translate, write and design. The group stopped talking about cognitive rehabilitation and began to talk about their wishes and desires – the things that brought joy to their lives and made their hearts sing. *My Life, My Goals* (Innovations in Dementia, 2021) was the resource developed by and belonging to people with dementia.

You can read more about co-production in practice in *The Right to a Grand Day Out: a story of co-production* (Innovations in Dementia, 2020). Here, people with dementia reached a point that they could never have imagined at the beginning of the project (in this case protesting with banners at a public railway station!) because of co-production. They had some recommendations for positive co-production (p.26):

- Have a belief that keeps you focused on what you are doing. Ours was 'Everyone has a right to accessible transport'.
- Keep it simple! Don't use jargon. Explain ideas.
- It's good to have some encouragement – to keep us on track and give us ideas.
- Find someone you trust to help you with the practicalities but don't let them take over.

---

2 https://sites.google.com/exeter.ac.uk/great-cr/home

- Don't feel you have to accept what others say. Keep challenging each other.
- Payment to our group has enabled us to keep involved in this project. It acknowledges our work and contributions to the learning around co-production.

Like PPIE, 'co-production' is a word that is used more in research and services than in everyday life. There is a danger that co-production and PPIE are not really practised in the truest sense of the words – that they are tokenistic and people with dementia don't feel valued.

Beyond co-production? Developing an alternative research involvement framework

We have already given examples of how people with dementia are involved in research, at varying levels of engagement. Research participation, PPIE and co-production have been shown to offer interesting opportunities, increasing people's self-confidence. People report feeling valued and empowered and these approaches result in better quality and more relevant research, shaped by the people who matter.

It is clearly a good thing that these opportunities are multiplying, and positive partnerships are being built between the research community and people with dementia (although this of course relies on best practice being implemented and absolutely no tokenism – which people can spot a mile off!).

Yet in spite of the shift to co-production and PPIE in dementia research, the locus of power still lies in the academic world – usually with universities and academic researchers. It is they who choose the research topic or questions, who design the methodology, who oversee the process, who lead on the analysis and who write up the findings and conclusions. As one Pioneer put it: 'We are still contributing on other people's terms.' This power imbalance inevitably effects what we view as the 'evidence' about dementia. And it perpetuates the partial view that dementia is a problem to be solved, rather than the context of the lives of almost one million people in the UK.

Dissatisfaction is still being expressed by some people with dementia who feel 'used' by academic researchers; they have a perception that they have been brought in to bolster the fundability of a piece of research.

There is also a sense that research is not yet asking and investigating the right questions about the things that people with dementia consider to be important. And most people with dementia are disconnected from the world of research, not realizing that their personal knowledge and experience of living with dementia is research gold dust. Research knowledge, processes and outputs are inaccessible to them.

But is there a next step? Is it possible for people with dementia to be in control of their own research agendas? With the right support could people with dementia lead their own research enquiries? What would happen if they were in the driving seat of research?

DEEP (Dementia Engagement and Empowerment Project), a project under the UK Network of Dementia Voices, offers a real opportunity to test out what 'going beyond co-production' can mean for people with dementia. DEEP provides access to a network of over 80 involvement groups of people with dementia connected to each other across the UK – more than 1000 people with dementia. DEEP connects groups to each other to magnify the voices, hopes and intentions of people with dementia, and to share learning. The network is diverse, including groups in care homes, and is strongly rooted in people's local communities. Groups are often supported and enabled by a facilitator, sometimes paid, often not; many facilitators of groups are themselves people with dementia. A facilitator helps a group to work together without taking over: they support the group in different ways to help the group to achieve its goals and are an important ingredient in how the group works and feels (Innovations in Dementia, 2022).

Rights and values are at the heart of the work of the network, with groups encouraged to identify and speak out about issues that are important to them. DEEP is hosted by the community interest company, Innovations in Dementia, and is part of a broader programme of work called Dementia Voices. One of the aims of the Dementia Voices programme is that people with dementia can exercise ownership and control in ways that best suit them, and with the necessary support and enablement. This is not always an easy thing to achieve, especially as the experience and impact of dementia often contributes to real, or perceived, losses of power and control. DEEP is built on a range of shared values, including influence, rights, opportunities, respect and unity. By connecting with each other, people with dementia have become more confident to speak out, their expectations have increased and their combined voices have greater impact. This grassroots movement is built on huge reserves of wisdom, knowledge and experience (and humour!), and provides a strong and supportive landscape in which to start to explore alternative approaches to more traditional or dominant perspectives. By increasing knowledge, it is possible to shift where power is situated.

DEEP provides the potential for a new approach to research delivery that is *led by* people with dementia. Many groups had already been involved in research studies carried out by universities. But as DEEP has developed over the past ten years (since 2012), people with dementia have been starting to *act as* researchers (even if not defining themselves as such), for example by:

- Identifying research priorities –
  Example: the Dementia Policy Think Tank group have co-produced a report to the United Nations on Human Rights (Innovations in Dementia, 2017).
- Testing out different ways of collecting information –
  Example: the Face It Together (FIT) group in Bradford have used videos and 'walk the patch' techniques to collect evidence of how hard it is to use local buses.
- Analysing information and thinking about what it means –
  Example: the Scottish Dementia Alumni group in Glasgow have collected contributions from people with dementia to produce a booklet on sensory challenges (Houston, 2017).

As projects like these gathered pace over the years, we were keen to explore with DEEP groups how research knowledge could be acquired and applied in a way that felt relevant to people's own lives, rather than being purely driven by the academic research agenda – in other words, to develop an alternative research involvement framework, and perhaps a different view of what evidence is. We wanted to increase the skills and knowledge of people with dementia, put power in their hands and support them to lead their own research. Ownership and control of the research would be in the hands of people with dementia. It would build on the strength of the DEEP network, with many involvement groups of people with dementia looking for opportunities to get 'stuck into' a project – to learn together, to build skills together and to find out the answers to questions about dementia that concern them.

It was this rationale that formed the basis of the concept for Dementia Enquirers – to give people with dementia themselves a chance to undertake their own research into dementia, rather than just being participants in other people's research. Through the DEEP network, people with dementia could be supported to identify their own research priorities and plan and carry out their own research. People with dementia could be at the heart of their own research.

The broader intentions for Dementia Enquirers were as follows:

- Research priorities would be driven by people with dementia, based on issues that are important to them.
- Participating DEEP groups would have a strengthened focus for the work they do – either locally or nationally – and would acquire research skills and knowledge that they could use again.
- Power imbalances would be challenged or reversed, with academic researchers bringing their research expertise into the DEEP network, rather than people with dementia always giving their lived expertise to universities.
- We would learn something about dementia-accessible research methods.
- People with dementia would feel valued and more empowered in the work they do in their DEEP group. We hoped this would have knock-on effects in their daily lives as opportunities and confidence increased.
- We would learn lots of new things together that could be shared with the wider dementia research community and beyond.

A key point to make as we prepared to run the Dementia Enquirers programme is that the world of research felt very alien to most people with dementia.

But we carried with us a confidence that this move into the research world could be achieved. Our hope was that we could share this confidence with others. And we already had some experience from the project 'The Right to a Grand Day Out' (Innovations in Dementia, 2020) which explored co-production methods with people with dementia. As part of this, we asked people with dementia who were not engaged with research what they understood by the term 'co-production'; it is probably accurate to say they were not very warm towards this word.

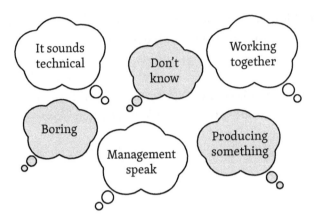

We used the issue of human rights to practise some co-production techniques in a project that became known as The Right to Get Out and About. But initially, when we asked people what they thought about rights, there was a resounding silence, just as there had been with the word 'co-production'! The *concept* of rights was not something that people were familiar with or interested in, and dementia rights felt far removed from people's lives.

So we started by thinking about rights in everyday life, about issues that felt relevant to people and close to home. The critical issue identified was transport. Transport can enable or disable us from getting out and about. Thinking about the right to get out and about made rights suddenly feel very real. During the project, 30 people with dementia actioned a project about social change and became more familiar with the idea of their rights and the rights agenda in general. There was so much interest in rights that the group made a trade union banner to march for their rights to get out and about!

The Right to Get Out and About concluded with three social action projects led by three groups of people with dementia. The Bradford Face It Together (FIT) group investigated the dementia accessibility of bus timetables; DEEP Vibes in Scarborough explored experiences of applying for Blue Badges; and York Minds and Voices considered the experiences of people with dementia travelling by train.

Each group:

- thought about topics of interest and importance to them
- set their research question

- described their rationale (why the topic was important)
- learned about a range of research methods
- went out into the field to collect data
- put it all together (their results)
- drew some conclusions
- made some recommendations.

In effect, they acted as researchers.

Sharing the driving seat

High-quality co-production (and PPIE) in research has got many benefits, according to people with dementia. True collaborations between people with dementia and researchers can result in:

- a range of expertise in the same place, with a balance of lived experience and researcher skills and knowledge
- opportunities for learning and development of new skills for people with dementia
- access to larger funding streams and therefore opportunities for more research.

Being in the driving seat

As you will read in this book, Dementia Enquirers has been about increasing the skills and knowledge of people with dementia to lead their own research. Their lived experience puts them in a very good position to say what dementia research should be about and how it should be carried out.

You will find out how people with dementia have adapted research methods and frameworks to be more dementia accessible, and have developed new ways of working within traditional research systems such as ethics processes. We hope you will see how people with dementia being in the driving seat of research really helps to make dementia research better. It is about shifting power and democratizing research. It doesn't mean that people with dementia have to do everything – but that they maintain the lead throughout.

CHAPTER 2

An Overview of the Programme

We decided to be Pioneers, because that is what we are doing – pioneering uncharted territory.

Chapter summary

In this chapter, we explain how and why the Dementia Enquirers programme took off, who was involved, the roles we took on, the connections and allies we made along the way, and the shifts in power that underpinned the programme. We also describe the many tangible outputs from the programme, including a suite of reports; accessible resources on research methods and ethics; a bespoke website; journal publications; book chapters; presentations and masterclasses; seminars and webinars; mini-internships with early careers researchers; and input into a university MSc course.

Funding

In 2018, and after many months of very constructive discussion, the National Lottery Community Fund (NLCF) awarded a large programme grant (£700,000) to Innovations in Dementia for a ground-breaking new initiative, Dementia Enquirers. The aim of the project (originally to be three-and-a-half-years, but extended to over four years because of the Covid-19 pandemic) was to develop a new approach to research, or 'enquiry', that is led and controlled by people with dementia themselves. We would support groups to identify research priorities and, helped by small grants, to plan and undertake their own research. The project would also explore with people with dementia the lessons that emerged from their work, and this learning would be widely shared. We were confident that the project could influence the prevailing approaches in research – while bringing new respect for the skills, expertise and resilience of those who are living with dementia.

By the end of the project we hoped that groups in the DEEP (Dementia Engagement and Empowerment Project) network would:

- have been supported to get better at research
- have enjoyed developing new skills
- feel more empowered and confident
- be better involved in other people's research
- have clear research priorities to share
- have encouraged the research community to work differently with people with dementia
- have some good ideas about more accessible ways of carrying out research.

The Pioneers

Very soon after we received the go-ahead from our funder, eight people with dementia came together to help to shape the programme. All were known to have a particular interest in research, all also brought with them a wide range of abilities and life experience – and all were highly motivated to make change happen:

> Why do we do it as Pioneers, why are we leading this work? That's about wanting change in the way research is carried out, and wanting change in the focus of research, so it's what matters to us. (George)

> More and more of us have said that we want to have ownership and control of the research. (Wendy)

The group chose the name of 'Pioneers'. As one of them explained:

> We did not really like the phrase 'Research Involvement Group'. Who's going to remember what a RIG is?! We've been bouncing ideas around about what to call our group, a name that properly describes our role to

help to steer this project. Pioneers? Board? Co-Leaders? Champions? We decided to be Pioneers, because that is what we are doing – pioneering uncharted territory.

The original Pioneers were:

Dr Wendy Mitchell
Rev. Mhari McLintock
Howard Gordon
Carol Fordyce
Teresa (Dory) Davies
Agnes Houston MBE
Tracey Shorthouse
Peter Berry

Carol and Peter were not able to stay in their roles for long because of other things happening in their lives. Mhari loved being a Pioneer, but eventually her worsening symptoms meant that she had to step down. Tracey was involved for several months before needing to step down too. Later, we were joined by George Rook – and, in Year 3, by Irene Donaldson, Steve Kennedy, Daithi Cee and Masood (Maq) Qureshi. These four were all suggested by the existing Pioneers, and were nominated not only to bring greater capacity to the group, but also to increase its diversity – in terms of ethnicity, sexual orientation and location.

The Pioneers have been given thank-you payments for their work at the NIHR/INVOLVE (National Institute for Health and Care Research / UK National Advisory Group) rate at £150 per day or pro rata, and have been supported throughout by Rachael Litherland and Philly Hare at Innovations in Dementia. They have influenced every single aspect of the programme – making every process more accessible, assessing grant applications and reflecting regularly on progress and learning.

Getting started

Our initial meetings were residential, giving us time to get to know each other and work at our own pace. We used two venues, one in London and one in Birmingham. Both were relaxing, calm environments with simple facilities and very helpful staff. This was more important to us than expensive but anonymous hotel facilities.

At the first programme meeting, in December 2018, a number of important decisions were made. The name and role of the Pioneers was agreed, as already explained, and a logo was selected.

We were adamant that processes would be kept as simple and accessible as possible. It was also decided that, instead of formal advisors, we would gather round us a small group of 'respectful friends or allies'. It was agreed that carers would not be invited into the Pioneers, as people with dementia needed to lead. But we would invite them as and when appropriate. In the event, carers have only been involved in order to support the person they are with.

We also came up with a wide range of ideas, many of which have been pursued:

- Produce a simple explanation of different methods.
- Produce guidelines for researchers.
- Update the guidelines for DEEP groups.
- Try to influence ethics committees.
- Use the National Lottery Community Fund philosophy of 'challenging the status quo'.
- Link local groups with local researchers.
- Link our work to human rights.

It is interesting to look back on some of the early quotes from the Pioneers which reflect their ambition and shared aspiration to do something really different:

> We have to prove we're capable.
> We have to be professional in all we do – we rise above any comments.
> We need to reflect our voices.
> We want to prove everyone wrong.
> It's got to be bottom-up.
> We need to make it a good process for everyone.

New projects are always exciting. You have an outline idea of what you hope to achieve, and some structure of how you think you will arrive at your destination. The rest comes from the work and energy of the project. However, Dementia Enquirers felt like an ambitious project – and there was some considerable fear! At the first meeting, the Pioneers expressed a number of concerns. Would academic researchers ask if they were really capable of doing research? Would they find using Zoom doable? Would the standard academic language be above them? As Carol, one of the Pioneers, said:

> I've got a tyre wrapped around my waist and I'm sinking!

But others were more optimistic:

> I'm energized... I'm happy.

> I've got a fear – but if not now, when? The thought of being able to be part of this really excites me. Maybe I can do something more academic... What an opportunity for us to influence things!

As the programme developed, the Pioneers grew in confidence. They took on many roles, including developing accessible application and selection processes; acting as ambassadors; presenting at events, webinars and conferences; co-authoring journal articles; making films; interviewing academics...and much more.

Early on, we also commissioned the cartoonist Tony Husband to create an image for us which really captured our aspirations and enthusiasm. (This image can be found on the Dementia Enquirers website.)

The arrival of the pandemic of course meant that we could only continue to meet online. Luckily, all of our Pioneers had Zoom skills, and for many this change did actually mean less fatigue from travelling to meetings. However, we all missed the lack of face-to-face contact and the social aspect of the residential meetings. Fortunately, we were able to re-instate these towards the end of the programme.

The roles of Innovations in Dementia staff

Dementia Enquirers has been hosted by Innovations in Dementia. Two of the co-directors – Rachael Litherland and Philly Hare, who have authored this book – have supported the programme throughout its duration, each committing six days per month. Rachael and Philly have been very flexible about their roles within the programme, though at times they have each focused on specific themes as they emerged. For example, Philly has tended to lead on the ethics work, and Rachael on the evaluation.

There has been a commitment throughout the programme for the Pioneers and staff to work together in every aspect. The principle which we applied at all times – or at least as far as we possibly could – was that the programme was guided by the people with dementia who were involved. We aimed to model what it means for people with dementia to be 'in the driving seat'. To achieve this, a lot of 'scaffolding' support was needed in the background, such as:

- applying for, and negotiating, funding
- recruiting and supporting the Pioneers
- making contact with advisors and other allies throughout the programme
- agreeing timelines to ensure objectives were met
- producing a regular newsletter, delivered to a mailing list that was steadily built up
- setting up the website (launched May 2021)
- commissioning a logo, and an image of people with dementia 'in the driving seat' (created by cartoonist Tony Husband)
- setting up/facilitating meetings and events, and drafting agendas
- recording and editing film footage
- managing social media
- managing enquiries
- reporting to the funder and negotiating an extension because of Covid-19
- developing an evaluation plan
- supporting and publishing the individual research projects
- co-producing resources
- encouraging reflection and feedback
- building partnerships
- co-delivering conference presentations and workshops.

Making connections and allies

As already mentioned, an early decision was made that, instead of recruiting formal advisors, we would gather round us a small group of 'respectful friends'. Whereas a formal advisory group might well have taken power away from the Pioneers, this model allowed them total control over how they made use of an informal network of experts.

The decision also freed the staff from the burden of producing formal agendas, minutes and so on, and allowed us to be more creative in how we recorded meetings (e.g. in the form of films).

Our key allies have included:

- Professor Dawn Brooker MBE (Worcester University)
- Dr David Crepaz-Keay (Mental Health Foundation)
- Professor Tom Shakespeare (London School of Hygiene and Tropical Medicine)
- Dr Rosie Ashworth (Partners in Research, Tayside NHS)
- Dr Lucy Series (Cardiff/Bristol Universities)

Although Tom, Dawn, Rosie, Lucy and David were our most regular and committed advisors, many others were involved at various points during the programme. Together they brought links with international networks and peer-reviewed journals, research expertise, knowledge of the literature, experience of mental health and disability service-user movements, expertise in law and ethics – and, most importantly, a commitment to the 'driving seat' philosophy.

One of the initial contributions of the advisors was to generate a feeling of real excitement and possibility. Here are some examples of the advice and encouragement they gave at the first meeting:

Advisors and other academics can take on some of the roles for you... but people with dementia must retain ownership.

If it looks too big and frightening, break it down and make it manageable.

Don't lose the excitement of why we're doing this. It is a transformative thing that we're trying to do. It's radical and progressive and needs to be done.

I want you to fly!

If you come across a 'charismatic idea'...it could be transformative. Be open to that.

You'll be a harmonious cacophony.

The advisors also gave some very practical initial advice. They suggested, for example, that we avoided projects involving the NHS because of the complex and time-consuming ethics requirements. They encouraged us to ensure our Pioneers group was as diverse as possible. They gave us 'permission' to broaden our vocabulary by using words such as 'enquiry' or 'storytelling' ('gentle language') and avoid narrow terms such as 'research'. They also reinforced the importance of being very clear about the question (what do you want to find out?), the audience (who do you want to influence?) and the method (how will you do it?).

The advisors were particularly helpful in balancing encouragement and reassurance with permission to be realistic:

> The fears are important to the whole project... You're ideally placed to keep us grounded...reining our enthusiasm back, to look at it in small chunks.

> Don't try to do everything – focus on original work and a few priorities – your USP. Match your ambitions to your resources and timescales. What is it in three years' time that you will be furious if you haven't done?

Working as equals – beyond 'patient and public involvement and engagement'

We wanted to make sure that this project made a difference, fired people up and added to what the world knew about dementia and dementia research. It also needed to be positive and enjoyable.

We wondered if even the word 'research' was off-putting. Our advisors helped us to think about this word. Research is basically the gathering of information to answer a question that is of interest to you. We might end up using other words to describe the work we do together – 'testimonials', 'storytelling' or (our very own) 'enquiry'.

We talked about the questions that interested us. We felt quite ambitious:

> We believed we could...and we did.

But we recognized that we needed to keep it simple, rein in our enthusiasm, stay grounded:

> If we're very clear about our outcomes, and go back from them, it's going to be more possible, less frightening – and we're all in this together, which made me feel good.

> Let's keep this simple. One step at a time.

> Make everything as simple as possible...but not simpler (paraphrase of a saying commonly attributed to Albert Einstein).

We also felt the pressure of time, which was quite motivating:

> I've got a fear – but if not now, when? The thought of being able to be part of this really excites me.

Making research methods accessible

At the very first meeting of the Pioneers and advisors, we recognized that, if people with dementia were to be in the driving seat of their own research, they would need accessible information and guidance about the most common research methods. We set about co-producing such a guide very quickly, and with great assistance from Dr Rosie Ashworth. It was published on our website in March 2019 as *How To Do a Research Project*, in time to inform our first round of grant applications – and was revised in 2023 (Innovations in Dementia, 2023a).

This guide tries to answer questions about all aspects of research. The reader is advised not to feel they have to read every page, as much of it will not be relevant to their research question. We designed it to be used as a manual – to be dipped into in search of an understandable answer to their questions. The sections are:

- Planning your project
- Ethics
- Consent forms
- Group discussions
- Interviews

- A survey (questionnaire)
- Listening to experts (Inquiry)
- Exploring the literature
- Evaluating an activity or service
- Outcome measures
- Needs assessments
- Visiting other places or services
- Writing your report
- Sharing what you have found out.

We have received a lot of positive feedback about this pack. For example, Professor Calum Davey, Deputy Director of the Centre for Evaluation at the London School of Hygiene and Tropical Medicine (LSHTM), commented:

> This handbook...is amazing. Must have been hugely challenging to write so clearly. Would recommend to anyone getting started (or teaching) research methods.

And as Agnes, one of the Pioneers, put it:

> Knowledge is power, and there's no point in having a good idea, if you don't know how to drive it forward. I think this [the research pack] is going to be one of the most powerful tools for me...

Making the funding and selection processes accessible

At the heart of this programme are the small research projects carried out by people with dementia themselves 'in the driving seat'. Throughout the four years, the Pioneers selected and gave grants to numerous small projects, all led by people with dementia themselves in their DEEP groups. As with everything else, the programme was severely affected by the pandemic. However, we are proud that we found ways to adjust and keep going, delivering three cohorts of projects (26 in total).

For each of the three cohorts, we together devised an accessible application and selection process. Once they had their grants, each project was linked to either Rachael or Philly, who kept in touch with them throughout. Some needed little support, others more. We relied on them to ask for what they needed as they were in the lead, but we were available to guide and troubleshoot if necessary. The final report of each project was formatted and designed, and then published on the website, starting with the first seven in May 2020.

You can find out more about the individual projects in Chapters 3 and 4.

Making ethics accessible

From our very first meeting, the topic of research ethics (and in particular, ethics approval processes) came up in discussion. It was seen by the Pioneers and advisors alike as potentially a major obstacle to people with dementia being 'in the driving seat'. It was proving very hard to find accessible information about the processes we might need to access.

By summer 2019, we had decided that we needed to co-produce an 'ethical framework' which was more tailored to research involving and/or led by people with dementia. *The DEEP-Ethics Gold Standards* was published in Summer 2020 (later revised and renamed *The Dementia Enquirers Gold Standards for Ethical Research*) (Innovations in Dementia, 2023b)

You can read more about this stream of work in Chapter 5. Again, we have received very positive feedback on this work on social media:

Tom Shakespeare @TommyShakes
I love working with @Innov_Dementia @DementiaVoices – I think this meeting may have just revolutionized the ethics of dementia research!

Bob Laventure @boblaventure4
Must be a better way, have met so many people frustrated and hindered in important and much-needed work.

James Rupert Fletcher @JamesRuFletcher
A really important issue. Procedural ethics can be a major impediment to dementia research. If this initiative develops and deals with the legal implications it could have a huge positive impact on the field.

James Rupert Fletcher @JamesRuFletcher
Replying to @WendyPMitchell @TNLComFund and 2 others
It's a big challenge but if anybody can do it you can! And it will test how truthful institutions really are when they say they value user involvement.

Rosie Ashworth @DrRAshworth
Over the last few days there has been such interest and excitement around the work of #DementiaEnquirers. It is so rewarding to see people come together to share in a common goal of supporting ethics committees to be more inclusive.

Sharing our learning

During the programme, we have co-produced a range of articles, which include:

- 'Dementia Enquirers – People with Dementia in the Driving Seat of Research' – an article for the peer-reviewed journal *Dementia* (Berry *et al.*, 2019).
- 'Dementia Enquirers: Pioneering Approaches to Dementia Research in the UK' – an article published in *Disability and Society* (Davies *et al.*, 2021).

We have also delivered a number of talks, webinars and conference presentations (see Appendix 3). These have mostly been online due to the global pandemic. In order to bring to the fore the voices of the people with dementia, these have almost always involved at least one of the Pioneers and/or film footage of others speaking.

The first event was a webinar on 'Dementia and Disability – connecting our worlds',[1] which we held in December 2019 on International Disabled People's Day. The webinar addressed the question: 'Leading our own research – what can people with dementia and people from other disability movements learn from each other?' It was hosted by LSHTM's International Centre for Evidence in Disability, in partnership with

---

1 https://soundcloud.com/dementia-diaries/dementia-enquirers-podcast-2-december-2019

Innovations in Dementia, and chaired by Professor Tom Shakespeare. The aim was to identify what people with dementia and their allies can learn from other disability movements (with particular regard to research) – and vice versa. The 15 or so invited delegates comprised the Pioneers alongside those with knowledge of different movements that have achieved (or want to achieve) change via research (e.g. movements of people with physical disabilities, learning disabilities, mental health issues). It was an opportunity for people working in different disciplines or movements to share ideas and knowledge about conducting disability research. We focused in particular on research that acknowledges the social model of disability, within the context of emancipatory research – research that is accountable to disabled people and is about social change.

Here are some of the key points to come out of the seminar:

- Self-advocacy groups are integral to developing inclusive research.
- Mental health survivor-led research has done much to change the nature of evidence – shifting what was considered to be knowledge and evidence away from just psychiatry.
- Colonization by academics is a risk; some are better at balancing than others.
- Questions to ask: (a) Who decided the research question? (b) Who decided what approaches to use? (c) Who controls the purse strings? (d) Who will be listed as co-authors?
- Some barriers in universities can be that co-writing takes longer, and usually happens at the end of a project.
- Even within co-production, hierarchies exist. Co-production is a process, not just an outcome. It's an aspiration to work in equal partnership even if hierarchies do exist.
- Lots of disability research is in development and a lot is unpublished. It is important to bring the results of co-produced research to journals.
- Research on public service reform doesn't tend to hit academic journals.
- It is a general challenge to academics to get out more and to know the best ways of involving people, and for research to be informed by lived experience.

- We need to think about power in the context of co-production. Some people don't want to hold the purse strings. It takes a long time.
- In dementia, there are challenges to involving people with more advanced dementia.
- Maybe we don't have to think about representativeness. There is a place for everybody.

In February 2020, we also held a seminar in London to discuss research ethics. You can read more about this in Chapter 5.

As part of the legacy plan for Dementia Enquirers, early career researchers from across the UK were invited in 2022 to apply for one of five mini-internships. To keep the application and selection processes as simple and accessible as possible, they were asked to send a two-minute video, which would be viewed by a selection panel of Pioneers. After watching these, the Pioneers selected seven successful applicants, each of whom were given a personalized session during May/June 2022, where they could focus on what *they* wanted to learn from the Pioneers. Both successful and unsuccessful applicants were also invited to a master-class in May 2022.

In Summer 2022, we were very pleased to start working with the University of Stirling to support them in integrating our *Dementia Enquirers Gold Standards for Ethical Research* into their online MSc course, the largest in the world. The Pioneers started the process by delivering an online session explaining their perspectives on research ethics and processes. They then responded to issues raised on the 'discussion board', as the students began to integrate the Standards into their project assignments. Finally, the students fed back to the Pioneers on how the Standards had influenced their thinking. This work has led on to another project with the University of Stirling, started in 2023, in which people with dementia are co-designing a new course for non-dementia specialists.

The impact of the masterclasses and mini-internships is discussed in more detail in Chapter 7.

Regular recording of reflections and conversations

Throughout the whole period of the programme, we held regular conversations and discussions. Some of these involved the Pioneers only, and others included some of our advisors. They were lightly edited and made into short films or podcasts.

We have also produced a range of leaflets and guides, all of which can be found on the Dementia Enquirers' website.[2]

---

2   https://dementiaenquirers.org.uk

CHAPTER 3

The Dementia Enquirers Projects

I do research because it's 'catnip to the brain'. I see it as a virtuous circle; me helping in the 'here and now' helps others in the future. What more could I ask for? (Martin)

Chapter summary

The only way that we were going to learn about people with dementia being 'in the driving seat' of research was to give it a go! At the heart of Dementia Enquirers was funding for a range of small research projects, which encouraged – indeed expected – DEEP (Dementia Engagement and Empowerment Project) groups to:

- decide what issues they were interested in exploring (a goal)
- identify a research question
- decide which methods or research approach they would take to answer their question
- collect data
- analyse the data
- report results
- think about conclusions
- acknowledge limitations
- make recommendations.

In essence, we invited them to lead and deliver research projects following the same framework as most other research projects.

In this chapter, we describe how we co-designed our application processes to be as accessible as possible, the successful projects which were selected and the topics they covered.

Selecting successful projects

We organized three funding rounds within the Dementia Enquirers programme:

Funding round 1	Ten projects	July 2019
Funding round 2	Five Covid-19-related projects	November 2020
Funding round 3	Eleven projects	August 2021

This chapter describes the process of selecting the 26 projects and gives a flavour of their different approaches to research. A fuller description of the projects can be found in Appendix 1. Chapter 4 will reflect on some of the processes involved in these projects.

Deciding what to fund

The Pioneers were in the driving seat when it came to deciding which projects to fund. In funding round 1, they met face-to-face as a decision panel. In funding rounds 2 and 3, the decision panel took place online, using Zoom. This was predominantly due to the Covid-19 pandemic and the longer-term shift away from face-to-face working.

In each round, all DEEP groups were invited to apply for a grant from Dementia Enquirers via a written application form. The application form was designed to be as short and accessible as possible. There were some guidance notes that could help people to complete their application. People could also phone Rachael or Philly for help to think about their application and the best way to put their ideas down on paper. The hope was that a range of groups would apply for the funding, and that we could help groups to feel more confident if they were feeling doubtful.

The Pioneers did not have to prepare for the decision-making panel, but they knew the agenda, the intended process and what to do in the event of a conflict of interest. This is the information they were given beforehand:

Process for making decisions about grants

- The decision-making panel is made up of the Pioneers group (six people with dementia).
- Philly and Rachael will act as *advisors* to the panel. They will not have voting rights. They can offer context, answer questions and raise any issues/concerns they think Pioneers should be aware of.
- Each application will have an *accessible summary* (written by Philly/Rachael) and this will be used to help with discussions. The summary will include:
  - the project title
  - project description
  - how people with dementia are in the driving seat
  - the research methods that have been chosen.
- The name and location of the group will be deleted.
- The main application forms will be available on the day for the panel to refer back to (with identifying features removed).
- Philly or Rachael will introduce each application using the accessible summary.
- Everyone will have a chance to talk together about the application and ask questions.
- We will each fill in a worksheet for each application and then compare our individual decisions. This worksheet has been designed around the criteria we have set for the funding. You need to respond to each question by choosing a face that best represents how you feel.
- 'Yes's and 'no's will be stacked in different piles. There will also be a 'not sure' pile.
- We will talk about the applications in the 'not sure' pile and try to move them to the 'yes' or 'no' pile.
- If there are too many applications in the 'yes' pile we will need to reduce them. We will display a large poster version of our Dementia Enquirers postcard – and ask the question, *Does this project really put people with dementia in the driving seat?* With numbered tokens, Pioneers will

individually place each project in a part of the poster (in the driving seat, being pulled behind or somewhere in between).

- You may have some outstanding questions about some applications. We can put these to one side and ask our advisors to help answer them.
- After you have decided on your preferred projects, Rachael will send our list to the National Lottery Community Fund (NLCF). This money is their money.
- With your list, you are *recommending* the projects that you would like to be funded. However, the NLCF will make the decisions. Rachael will also send them some notes of our meeting.
- We will let you know the decisions of the National Lottery Community Fund.

Conflicts of interest

- A Pioneer may be a member of a DEEP group that has applied for a grant. These applications will be considered at the end.
- A Pioneer linked to the application will not be able to comment or vote on their particular application.
- Other Pioneers will need to be professional and not influenced by their relationship with the linked Pioneer.

Summaries of the applications were made by Rachael and Philly, with any identifying information removed to avoid bias. The summaries turned the applications into bullet points and removed any extraneous words. Score sheets were created and we practised with them beforehand. At this point, we realized that a scale of numbers and even smiley faces doesn't work for everyone. The Pioneers added words that captured the meaning of the numbers and faces: (1) super-sad (2) sad (3) fine/OK/neutral/so-so (4) happy (5) super-happy. In practice, we also sometimes used facial expressions and movement to indicate our feelings and scores. For one Pioneer an excited dance movement indicated a (5) – super-happy!

Table 3.1: Score sheet for grant applications

Application number:
You can use this scale to answer the following questions:

	Your score	Please explain your answer
How does the research question make you feel?		
Do you feel that people with dementia have been or will be in the driving seat?		
How appropriate are the methods the group has chosen?		
How much difference will this project make to the group, to DEEP and to the world?		
How ethical does this project feel to you?		
Any other comments?		

In the funding rounds 2 and 3, the decision-making panel moved online due to Covid-19 and the restrictions this brought. Online meetings are very tiring for people with dementia, and so we ran a number of meetings over an entire week – 90 minutes each and making decisions on two or three applications per day.

The Projects

Before we move on to describe the different projects that were funded by Dementia Enquirers, it is worth noting the variety of topics that groups decided to research. They were very diverse and driven by the interests of each different DEEP group. And they were usually the subjects that groups regularly discussed or were uppermost in their minds as the funding became available. And they were the issues that people with dementia identified as important.

The projects were usually small in scale and mostly used qualitative research methods or surveys. Our advice was to take a simple idea and use research methods to try and find out some answers. We did not want groups to be 'put off' at the first hurdle. DEEP groups were not researchers to begin with – but they became researchers! In the first instance, though, we were clear that the grants were for groups of ordinary people with dementia who wanted to find out the answer to a question.

In Chapter 6, read about our work around accessible research processes.

List of the successful projects

THRED in Liverpool (Project 1)
THRED explored how urban and rural transport systems can help people with dementia to live independently for longer.

Minds and Voices in York
Minds and Voices looked at the benefits, challenges and different experiences of people living alone with dementia compared to those who lived with a care partner.

Beth Johnson Foundation in Stoke-on-Trent (Project 1)

This group looked at whether class, intellect or ethnicity had an impact on dementia pathways for the person with dementia.

Riversiders in Shrewsbury and Minds and Voices in York

These groups explored what DEEP group members and Admiral Nurses know about each other. (Admiral Nurses are specialist dementia nurses who are supported and developed by Dementia UK.)

Our Voice Matters in Hartlepool

This group looked at the impact of community-based groups on people with dementia.

Deepness on the Isle of Lewis

Deepness looked at what type of video content works best for people with dementia.

EDUCATE in Stockport

This project explored how people with dementia used Alexa (Amazon Echo Dot), and what benefits or difficulties they experienced.

SHINDIG in Sheffield

This looked at the practical and psychological impact of having to give up driving because of dementia.

SUNShiners in Dover, Deal and Shepway

SUNShiners investigated what the public knew about dementia, including what they thought about the invisibility of dementia.

STAND in Fife

This project asked people with dementia what they thought the new Fife Dementia Strategy should include.

THRED in Liverpool (Project 2)

This explored the transport-related hopes and fears of people with dementia during and after Covid-19.

Budding Friends in Exeter
This project explored the impact of Covid-19 on the physical and mental wellbeing of people with dementia.

Forget-me-nots in Canterbury
This project looked at how Covid-19 had affected people with dementia in Kent in relation to technology, relationships, coping and physical and mental health.

Beth Johnson Foundation in Stoke-on-Trent (Project 2)
This group explored how people with dementia managed during the Covid-19 pandemic.

Riversiders in Shrewsbury
This group carried out a survey of people with dementia to find out if they were offered an annual dementia review by their GP and, if they were, whether or not they found it helpful.

Scottish Dementia Alumni in Scotland
This group developed a game for children to help them understand dementia.

ECREDibles in Scotland
This was a new partnership between people with dementia and the Edinburgh Centre for Research on the Experience of Dementia (ECRED) team at Edinburgh University. The aim of this project was to find out how a group of people living with dementia could work in partnership with a university project in order to lead research.

Forget Me Not Centre in Swindon
This project explored people's experiences of post-diagnostic support and ideas for improving practice.

Lifting the Cloud in Derby
This group visited and researched various visitor attractions in Derby, investigating what it was like to visit as a person with dementia.

Up and Go in Leeds

This group conducted a survey to find out whether a dementia diagnosis can open doors to new opportunities.

Ashford Phoenix in Kent

This group wanted to find out whether people with dementia benefitted more from learning a new musical instrument, rather than just being participants in music sessions.

Beth Johnson Foundation in Stoke-on-Trent (Project 3)

This group explored different people's experiences of dementia testing. They were interested in consistencies and inconsistencies.

Great Camden Minds in London

This project explored how easy it is to find printed information about dementia services in Camden.

THRED in Liverpool (Project 3)

This group investigated barriers to people with dementia when travelling on public transport and the things that might encourage people to travel by public transport more often.

Switchboard Collaboration

This project aimed to understand the experiences of non-binary individuals with dementia.

You can read more detail about these projects in Appendix 1. The full reports, compiled and written by the different groups, are a must-read.[1] You will see that all the projects are very different in the way they were designed, delivered and written about.

Surveys, interviews and focus groups were common methods in many of the projects. But some groups did things a bit differently, and there was a lot of learning by doing. This can be described as action research. For example, Scottish Dementia Alumni created a new game (and encouraged learning) through trials with people with dementia.

---

1   https://dementiaenquirers.org.uk/individual-projects

Lifting the Cloud in Derby carried out dementia audits and therefore learned a lot via action research. EDUCATE in Stockport distributed Alexa devices to members with dementia, who first learned how to use them and then provided data about how they worked and felt in practice. Ashford Phoenix even learned to play ukuleles (rather successfully!) and measured their experiences over time.

What all projects do have in common, however, is that they start at the very beginning of a standard research ladder. The research proposals that were put forward were all based on issues that the group identified as *important to them* to explore. Even in high-quality research co-production, people with dementia do not usually get involved until after the research question and methodology have been decided.

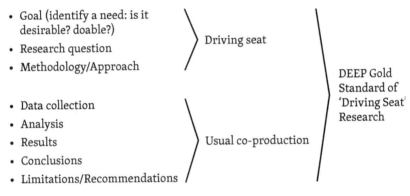

- Goal (identify a need: is it desirable? doable?)
- Research question
- Methodology/Approach

Driving seat

- Data collection
- Analysis
- Results
- Conclusions
- Limitations/Recommendations

Usual co-production

DEEP Gold Standard of 'Driving Seat' Research

DEMENTIA ENQUIRERS RESEARCH LADDER

Later in this book, as we build a Dementia Enquirers model of research in practice, we will explore just how important (and unique) it is for people with dementia to be involved at the very start of the research process.

CHAPTER 4

Opening up the World of Research

We have the expertise, but you provide the scaffolding.
We have the key, you can help us to open the box.

Chapter summary

This chapter describes the ways in which we made the world of research more accessible. We explain the values, the 'scaffolding' and the reasonable adjustments that underpinned the 26 projects and the Dementia Enquirers programme as a whole. We share information about accessible research methods and processes and discuss the impact of taking this approach. Much of this has been learned, built on and honed along the way. We also set out some recommendations for supporting people with dementia to be involved in research as co-producers.

Moving into research

From earlier work with the DEEP (Dementia Engagement and Empowerment Project) network we knew that some groups of people with dementia wanted to get involved in projects that they had conceived and then delivered. These have included art projects, poetry writing, learning photography, delivering dementia awareness sessions and carrying out dementia-accessible audits. Moving into research felt like a positive next step, especially in light of the criticisms from people with dementia about the (often tokenistic) way the research community engaged with them.

However, as we have also explained in Chapter 1, such an ambitious programme could mean that people ended up feeling outside their comfort zones. Remember Carol and that tyre around her waist causing her to sink? At the start of the first cohort of projects we asked people with dementia whether they felt like researchers. The answer was a resounding 'no'!

At the end of each round of grants we gathered groups together to reflect on their work. In discussing the impact of taking part in their Dementia Enquirers project, it was here that people with dementia began to identify as researchers.

> I've learnt a lot. I am happy. It has been a journey. (Up and Go group member)

> We're exhausted. But we achieved what we set out to do. (Ashford Phoenix group member)

> We took part as equals. Being researchers has given us energy. (ECRED-ibles group member)

> We did the work. Our facilitators helped with the sat nav. But we did the driving! (Beth Johnson Foundation group member)

So what were the elements that caused this shift in perspective as people with dementia took on identities as researchers?

Changing the language

We've already mentioned how overwhelming it can feel to be 'in the driving seat' of research. For many people, even the word 'research' caused some worries:

> Research is full of academic language – is it going to be above me? (Dory)

Wendy, who had worked with researchers, felt they would question the capabilities of people with dementia, and suggest that they couldn't or shouldn't be involved in research. However, she immediately countered this perspective by saying:

> But it's an opportunity to amaze people with what we can do. (Wendy)

Mhari acknowledged Carol's fear, but wanted to rise above it:

> I've got a fear, but if not now, when? The thought of being part of this really excites me. Maybe I *can* do something more academic. What an opportunity to influence things. (Mhari)

One of the first things we did was to change the way we talked about research. We began by asking people what the word 'research' meant to them. Here are some responses:

- scary
- medical
- something that happens in universities
- complicated
- full of jargon
- does things to us – it's distant to us.

Some of these ideas about research might have contributed to the fears described above. We focused on a simple definition of research as an activity that involves finding out things you do not know or trying to answer a question that you are interested in. It was then very easy to think about the important research questions. Here is the list the Pioneers came up with about the topics that interested them:

- What coping strategies and solutions do people with dementia have for living with dementia?
- What do people with dementia think about death (hospices, counselling)?
- How can people with dementia get the most out of mainstream technology such as apps and Alexa?
- What is known about hyperacusis (reduced tolerance of sound) and dementia?
- What imaginative uses do people with dementia have for Direct Payments (i.e. payments from your Council which let you choose and buy the services you need yourself)?
- What are people with dementia's experiences of benefits and money?

- What is the effect of relationships with carers and families on the person with dementia?
- What examples are there of self-management?
- How can services personalize communication with people with dementia?
- What perceptions are there in society today about dementia?
- What kind of funding for dementia do GPs receive and how do they use it?

We began to think about 'questions we want to know the answers to' rather than 'research'. Our advisors also suggested we use gentler language to begin with, e.g. enquiry, storytelling, testimonies. With a list of ideas and a broadened vocabulary, our fears began to quieten down!

Deciding what to research

We advised the DEEP groups that were applying to us for small grants to choose their research topic by thinking about what would help themselves and others – but also what they felt passionate about. We also suggested that their topic should be something that hadn't been researched much before (or at least be something to which they could bring a new perspective).

It was important that their research applied 'good' research processes. Our task was to make the world of research understandable to people who did not have much experience of doing it, at least in this format.

We found that this opening task was not difficult for DEEP groups. They had usually been discussing the issues that concerned them for a long time. Each group had different priorities and interests, and this is reflected in the range of Dementia Enquirers projects that were funded.

Starting the research

Research can often feel big and scary. Our academic advisors reassured us that all researchers feel like this when starting out:

> You're starting with a big ball of clay, but don't be afraid that you won't get a pot out of it at the end. Your lovely thing will evolve! (Professor Dawn Brooker MBE)

But there are some things to be clear about:

- The question – what do you want to find out?
- The audience – who do you want to influence?

Answers to these points determine the best methods to carry out research. Different approaches impress different people and help to prove to people that your conclusions are soundly based.

Choosing a research method

The choice of research method should be the one that is most useful in helping people find the answers to their questions. However, there is also a reality check – do you have the skills to apply your chosen method? If the answer is 'no', then you may need some other help from people who do know.

As we were reminded by one of our advisors, it's OK to ask for help:

> It's very unusual to carry out a research project in complete isolation. As an academic researcher, I might need help with statistics or someone to also look at my interpretations of interview data. A team of people makes the research better. I couldn't do it alone. (Professor Tom Shakespeare)

There are many research methods available to choose from: question-naires, interviews, focus groups, randomized controlled trials. People could also choose to carry out an enquiry, evaluation, observation or needs assessment. They might visit other places or services to compare it to the one under investigation. The Dementia Enquirers resource *How To Do a Research Project* (Innovations in Dementia, 2023a) described all of these research methods and helped groups to think about the best one to answer the questions they wanted to explore.

Perhaps not surprisingly, most of the Dementia Enquirers projects decided to use interviews, focus groups or questionnaires to gather their data. These were methods that people were familiar with from other areas of life, and many had experience of being on the other side of their use (i.e. as a research participant).

Case study: York Minds and Voices

People with dementia from York Minds and Voices carried out five individual interviews and one group interview. They wanted to find out about the experiences of people with dementia who lived alone, compared to those who lived with a care partner.

Beforehand, people from Minds and Voices agreed an approach about how they were going to run the interviews. They asked the group facilitator to be in charge of some of the research protocols. This included organizing the Zoom meetings and going through a consent process with the interviewees, which reduced some of the administrative burden for group members. The interviewers with dementia agreed the format of each interview, consistency in how the questions would be asked and the importance of confidentiality and anonymity. Interviewees were sent the interview questions beforehand to allow them to prepare, including being able to write down comments that they might want to make. There was an empathy from the interviewers with dementia about how stressful and distracting it can be to be asked interview questions without being able to remember what you want to say. After the interviews had been carried out the interviewees reflected that the shared experience of dementia had built a quicker rapport between interviewer and interviewee. There was a strong (and instant) sense of trust between people and idea that the interviewer could 'get to parts that other people couldn't reach' because of a shared experience of dementia.

Values

Values are basic and fundamental beliefs that guide or motivate attitudes or actions. They help us to determine what is important. The values at the heart of the DEEP network had already been agreed:

- Unity – DEEP is a place where we come together as part of a network of groups.
- Opportunity to have a voice – DEEP provides equal opportunities for all voices in our groups to be heard and involved, and contribute about what matters to us.
- Respect – DEEP members respect different views and voices.

- Our voices – DEEP is about more than one voice; it is a powerful, collective network.
- Busting the stigma of dementia – DEEP members respectfully challenge the stigma of dementia through our voices and our activities.
- Influence – DEEP members can aim for any level of influence in the dementia world: your home, your street, your country. No action is too small.
- Honesty – DEEP offers a safe place to be raw, emotional and even angry, while being respectful and mindful of the needs of others.
- Love – DEEP groups encompass a sense of safety, belonging and unity.
- Humanity – DEEP members treat each other with kindness and respect.
- Anchor – DEEP provides a safe environment to belong and enable.

Dementia Enquirers practises all the DEEP values, as well as focusing very firmly on shifting the place where power is situated, in this case in relation to research. We believe that this continuity in the value base helped DEEP members to move across into the research world.

Values can feel hard to live by. For academic researchers, values might not be something they have really thought about in relation to their work. But in engaging more equally with people with dementia these are some of the ways these values can play out in research practice:

- Leadership – enabling, not dictating; providing the 'scaffolding'.
- Valuing everyone (and ourselves). It's the person that matters.
- Treating people with dementia as equals/partners – sharing power.
- Creating trust.
- Encouraging/enabling growth, confidence and self-belief.
- Recognizing everyone's experience and knowledge – don't exclude.
- Flexibility – willingness to do things differently.
- Safety – for each person, not one-size-fits-all.
- Clarity (no acronyms, jargon).

- Smiles! Warmth.
- Determination/passion to make change happen and overcome difficulties.
- Perseverance, strength, willingness to challenge.
- Liberation from rigidity, from the spider's web, from the academic walls.
- Humility and openness.
- Learning by doing.
- Teamwork – acceptance of each other's skills.

(Taken from a Pioneers residential event, October 2022.)

Scaffolding

People with dementia have described an importance of the *support* that has enabled them to become dementia researchers. This is highlighted by people with dementia within projects as well as the Pioneers who help to shape the whole Dementia Enquirers programme.

We are probably most familiar with scaffolding as a raised structure that supports workers and materials during a building project. It is also a term used in education, where it means providing a particular kind of support to students as they learn or develop a new concept or skill, with the teacher stepping back as the student becomes more confident. In Dementia Enquirers, people with dementia described scaffolding as 'invisible support', there in the background giving practical help, 'geeing us up and enabling us to shine' (Chris, Ashford Phoenix).

This is how the Pioneers have defined scaffolding:

- mentoring and support
- adjustments to how we work
- buy-in to DEEP values
- negotiation and flexibility
- behind the scenes support – administration
- looking after us, taking the strain off us
- keeping contact, arranging meetings, managing us
- high expectations of us – but realistic
- making systems work for us.

In various ways, other people have provided the scaffolding that has supported people with dementia in DEEP groups to learn new skills and to 'shine' as researchers. This has often been a DEEP group facilitator:

- providing administrative support – setting up meetings, organizing interviews, printing out surveys and accompanying project materials
- supporting people directly in some of the research tasks where needed. See Brian's case study below for an example of carrying out a literature review
- keeping in mind the original project proposal, and being able to support the group to return to their original objectives when the research ideas grow and change
- holding the views of the group in the research development phase, and reflecting this back to the group to consider
- reminding the group where they have got to in their project
- transcribing interviews
- writing down the final report with and on behalf of the group
- motivating everyone, especially at the bit of the research process when everything feels impossible
- oiling the creative juices with whatever it takes (tea and biscuits!).

Providing scaffolding rather than taking the lead is not always easy! As Dani from SUNShiners said:

It was a challenge sometimes. I needed to step back and bite my tongue. We had collected so much data to analyse. It was far too overwhelming. A lot of what we did next was trial and error and meeting in the middle.

Reasonable adjustments that help people with dementia in research

People with dementia have identified a number of practical adjustments that help them to be involved in research:

- Start from the assumption that people with dementia CAN.
- Don't use research jargon. Find more familiar words that get across the ideas.

- Recap on previous meetings and conversations. Provide a summary of what happened previously.
- Reinforce words with pictures and images.
- Keep meetings short. Make sure there are refreshments and breaks. Research involves a lot of concentration.
- Make sure the research is worth doing. Nobody wants their time wasted. Research questions developed by or with people with dementia help to make sure the research is worth doing.
- Encourage turn-taking in research discussions. Use the 'I Want to Speak' card[1] to make sure that people can speak when they need to.
- Ensure the environment is conducive to research, for example in safe, private spaces.
- Make sure the time of day for research is the best for the person. Some people are better in the mornings, other people in the afternoons. Find out what's best for people.
- Be aware and open about the fact that some topics are emotional. This does not mean you should avoid them, but give some thought to how you can create a safe emotional space.
- Use props, pictures, tools such as Talking Mats and easy-read information to help people take on research roles. Avoid overloading people with information.

A note about capacity

Very few people with dementia do research on their own – if they do, they will doubtless have capacity to do so. If part of a team, it is still possible for a person 'without capacity' to contribute. This is the case in many activities undertaken by DEEP groups. For example, they may have skills in illustrating. They could offer themselves as guinea pigs for testing interview schedules. They can help to develop themes for exploration by contributing their own experiences.

Now let's look at some ways in which people with dementia were in the driving seat of their Dementia Enquirers projects.

---

1 www.dementiavoices.org.uk/wp-content/uploads/2021/11/I-want-to-speak-card-english.pdf

Carrying out a literature review – Brian

Finding out what other researchers have previously learned is an important first step to carrying out your own research. You want to know how your project might be different and what it could add to what is known about the subject. Or as Brian said: 'We could look what's on t'internet!'

Eight articles about living alone or with a care partner were identified. These were verbally summarized for Brian. They covered:

- experience of loss and relationship quality in couples
- living with a partner with dementia: lived experiences of changes
- the significance of the home as perceived by people with dementia
- exploring neighbourhood connections for people living alone with dementia
- expression of togetherness in couples
- living alone with dementia: findings from the IDEAL (University of Exeter) cohort
- shared experience of humour
- precarity of older adults living alone with cognitive impairment.

The literature review revealed a gap in more clearly being able to identify the benefits, challenges and different needs of people living alone and people living with a partner. This knowledge paved the way for the York Minds and Voices project.

Carrying out our research: supportive allies who were good at admin – Forget-me-nots, Canterbury

Additional to the working party of people with dementia were placement psychology students and volunteers. They would help to set up virtual meetings, keep notes and help to chair meetings.

Themes for questions were developed in the working party, and then the students and volunteers contacted other people with dementia in the Forget-me-nots group to discover their thoughts and opinions about the question themes. The questions to be asked in the survey were redrafted based on this information.

Students or volunteers ensured that the consent forms were filled in and they set up the online interviews at a mutually convenient time. A student or volunteer attended the meeting to support each person with dementia to access the meeting. But they played little or no role in the interview itself. Once the interviews were complete, the students and volunteers conducted informal transcription and thematic analysis to establish key points.

The group acknowledged that the students helped them to see considerable growth in their abilities and knowledge, by allowing the project to run very smoothly.

Helping people to prepare for their research participation – Forget Me Not Centre research group, Swindon

The researchers with dementia knew first-hand the stresses of being a research participant. They wanted to make their research process as supportive as possible.

The group designed a recruitment poster, acknowledging that the researchers were people with dementia. They thought this would level the research playing field. Once someone had got in touch and expressed an interest in taking part, they met each participant individually over Zoom to explain the study and gain consent to take part in focus groups.

They designed a simple booklet which had the four topics that would be covered in the focus groups. They did this so that people could prepare what they wanted to say if they wanted to and wouldn't feel 'on the spot'. They left space in the booklet for the participant to make notes under each topic. That way, if they forgot in the moment, they could refer to the booklet.

Choosing a measurement scale – Ashford Phoenix

The group wanted to use a validated measurement to measure the impact of their music sessions. They wanted to use a standardized scale so other organizations would recognize their work. They also wanted to include measures of people's mood as well as aspects of life with dementia. The group enlisted the help of Jack, an assistant psychologist.

Jack found the Brief Moods Introspection Scale (BMIS) (Mayer & Gaschke, 1988). The group decided this scale wasn't very dementia friendly given how jumbled it looked with statements and numbers. They agreed to swap the numbers on the measurement scale to faces, with a face put in place for each option.

The group also wanted room to express their wider thoughts on the music sessions, so extra space was included beneath each question for people to write down any thoughts or feelings.

A point about research ethics

We quickly realized that we had a lot of work to do on making ethics more accessible. You can read more about our work in this area in Chapter 5, including information about the Gold Standards we co-produced.

This thinking resulted in the following checklist, which was used as the Pioneers assessed the Dementia Enquirers project application forms.

Checklist for assessment of project proposals

☐ 1. Is it clear what is planned?
☐ 2. Have they thought about consent processes?
☐ 3. Have they mentioned a written information sheet?
☐ 4. Would it be possible to easily recognize the participants?
☐ 5. Will they discuss this with people?
☐ 6. Will they anonymize people if necessary?
☐ 7. Will they feed back to participants at the end of the project?
☐ 8. How accessible will the project materials be? (May be a worry if the application itself isn't very accessible.)
☐ 9. Does the project feel 'invasive'? If so, check more fully in the ethics Gold Standards.
☐ 10. Are people with dementia in the driving seat of this project?

Staying in the driving seat

The driving seat model has been mentioned early on in this book when we set out the rationale for what Dementia Enquirers has been trying to achieve. We will also explore it more completely in Chapter 8. A criterion for awarding a Dementia Enquirers grant to a project was that people with dementia were in the driving seat. 'Driving seat' is also assessed in the above form as an ethical issue (point 10).

But what do people with dementia understand by 'driving seat'? As with many research terms, it is one that we adopted with some logic at the start of the project (and on which we successfully acquired funding for the programme). But we soon found that it means different things to different people, particularly with regard to how it is put into practice.

This is what the 'driving seat' looked like after we had run the first round of grants. We created it in discussion with Pioneers and also people with dementia who had been part of the first cohort of grants. We understand that people with dementia will contribute at different levels and in different ways. But here are some things which show that you and your group are well on the way (we don't expect everyone to meet all of these):

- Everyone chooses and agrees the topic together.
- Everyone chooses the methods together.
- Everyone is involved in the project budget as much as they want to be.
- Everything is fully accessible – the language, the process, the venues etc.
- The group communicates, recaps and updates in a way that is most helpful to each individual (using very creative methods when needed).
- Everyone uses the skills they feel comfortable with, and as much as they wish.
- Everyone has the chance to learn new skills: 'It's about what you need, not just to stay the same, but to *grow*. Not needs-led or care-led, but *desire-led*.'
- People sometimes come to *your turf,* rather than you always going to theirs.
- Everyone shares in decision-making.
- Everyone says what support they need.
- Everyone is fully 'in the loop' (including receiving the Dementia Enquirers newsletter).
- Everyone understands what everyone's role is.
- Everyone feels 'in control'.
- Everyone feels safe and respected, and encouraged to contribute as they can.
- Everyone comes up with solutions to problems together.
- Everyone is able to have a 'buddy' to support and encourage them.
- Everyone is invited to connect with other groups, for example through Zoom.

'Driving seat' is a concept that is hard to pin down and even harder to measure! Perhaps it is easier to think about it as a thread running through a project. It is a feeling, a value and a principle – more noticeable when it is not there.

Some groups sought help for aspects of their research projects. This does not mean that they did not remain in the driving seat, in control and leading their research. But, as Tom Shakespeare noted, they drew on additional expertise where they identified a need for it. For example, facilitators carried out administrative tasks, such as setting up interview schedules, adding questionnaires to SurveyMonkey or writing a draft report based on guidance from the group. Other times the groups chose to commission the help that they needed. This is discussed further in Chapter 5. In Appendix 2, you can find a case study about how the SUNShiners group dealt with their large data set. We will return to the driving seat model in Chapter 8.

Writing up the research findings

The Dementia Enquirers projects almost all produced a final report.[2] We gave them some ideas about how to present their research in a report, following a fairly simple structure:

- Title (make sure it includes some key words)
- Names of authors
- Introduction (a summary of what the report is about and its structure)
- Background to the research – don't assume the reader knows anything about the subject
- Your research question and your aims
- What you did to collect information (your methods)
- A description of the research actions and their results
- Your conclusions
- List of references (including any other reports that have helped you with your findings)
- Acknowledgements (to thank those who have helped in any way)

---

2   https://dementiaenquirers.org.uk/individual-projects-dementiaenquirers

We suggested that the report could include quotes, case studies and photographs (with permission) to bring the human touch. We also recommended that people think about accessible formatting, such as:

- the font you use (Arial 14 point is a good one)
- how you space the lines (1.5 is good)
- using colour to differentiate
- including page numbers.

You can find out more about accessible writing by reading *How to Write and Produce Better Information for People with Dementia* (Innovations in Dementia, 2023c).

There was a variety of styles of writing in the final Dementia Enquirers reports. Some reports were written in their entirety by people with dementia. Others were created from group discussions, and some from dictation and a helping hand from people who didn't have dementia. But commonly the reports:

- included photos of the authors – a lovely variety of group photos in a variety of settings
- described how the research question had arisen
- described how the methods were decided on (a lot of creation seemed to occur in social venues such as the pub or with copious amounts of tea and cake!)
- kept the experiences of people with dementia at the heart of their writing
- avoided jargon, using language that was understandable to a lay audience
- set out what the group had gained from leading a research project.

Perhaps there are some ideas here that academic researchers could draw on when writing up their research for publication. People with dementia are very keen to know what the outcomes of research studies are, but they very often find that the reports or papers are inaccessible to them, either because of writing style or other barriers to access. Sharing what you have found out is an important part of the research cycle. Creative and accessible research reports and lay summaries can really help to communicate research findings as widely as possible.

Getting involved – or not – in Dementia Enquirers

What made some groups apply for the Dementia Enquirers funding, while others did not? There are around 80 groups in the DEEP network and we had 32 applications in total, across the three cohorts. These represented 27 groups (some groups made more than one application, and some applications involved more than one group).

From our feedback from those who did apply, it is clear that this was viewed as a great opportunity to do something they might not otherwise be able to do. In some cases, they were able to focus on topics that were very close to their hearts, issues such as giving up driving or annual GP assessments that they had been discussing for months or even years. In the case of the EDUCATE group, one member, Steve, had previously been involved in a European Union robotics project, testing a domiciliary 'care bot'. At the time, he questioned the value of spending millions on a robot when a lot of its functions could be carried out by Alexa. Steve's insight, combined with the funding from Dementia Enquirers, created the momentum leading to this enquiry.

Twenty-five per cent of DEEP groups applied to run a Dementia Enquirers project. It is not clear why many groups did *not* apply. The opportunity did not resonate with everyone. We know that some groups who would have liked to have carried out a project were limited by factors such as availability of support, commitments of the group and/ or their facilitators to other pieces of work, and lack of time and energy. We have previously acknowledged the fragility of DEEP groups (Litherland, 2015) which often rely on precarious local funding, committed facilitators with personal drive (whose circumstances or job roles can suddenly change), and high-quality, early diagnosis in the local area. Carrying out a piece of user-led research can be difficult to prioritize in these circumstances, even if the will is there. Some may have been put off by the terminology of research and not see it as something that they can do, as we know that the Pioneers were initially.

One project did not start, and a couple of others handed their funding back because of difficult personal circumstances for their group facilitator. However, we know that groups in our cohort 3 were inspired by what groups in the first cohort had achieved (and some groups returned for repeat funding as they had enjoyed the experience so much!). We suspect that, were Dementia Enquirers to continue, there would be greater uptake of the research grants, with earlier groups providing mentorship.

Recommendations for supporting people with dementia in co-research

We have learned so much in this programme about what is different in research led by people with dementia themselves. Clear, accessible communication is a crucial part of the 'driving seat' model. If language and processes are unclear, they are effectively *unethical*, because they exclude people and prevent them for contributing to their full potential. Here are some ways we can all help.

Explain your project

- Take time to find out each person's preferred ways of communication.
- Give enough information (but not too much) to enable people to make an informed decision about whether to take part.
- Keep everything as simple as possible – tailor your information so it is fit for purpose, for the audience and for the level of risk.
- Use photos and other images if this helps to convey information.
- Avoid overloading people with other (less accessible) information where it's not absolutely necessary.
- Give people enough time to ask questions and make decisions.

Obtain consent

- Offer extra help to give informed consent. Visual props, Talking Mats, easy-read information and so on can help people to understand and decide whether to be involved.
- If people cannot sign a form, allow them to record their agreement on video or audio, or you could write a 'field note'.
- Accept that consent is an ongoing and flexible process. Provide

routine reminders and recaps (verbal, written or pictorial) that prompt people to reconsider and reflect on their involvement.

Make participation easier

- Remind participants the day before that they will be meeting with you, using the communication method that they indicate is best for them.
- Offer to help with travel plans, remote access, meeting people at stations and so on, if they need/want this to keep them safe.
- Make the schedule flexible to people's preferred time of day, and avoid days where other support might be limited (e.g. Friday evenings).
- Ensure that the research is conducted in a quiet, safe, private space and is in keeping with the participant's wishes (if at all possible).
- For group discussions, think carefully about the venue – it needs to be peaceful, welcoming, fully accessible, well-signposted, with easy parking and transport links.
- Present all information clearly and accessibly, making reasonable adjustments as needed (including translation/interpretation). DEEP has provided guidance on writing accessible information for people with dementia.[3]
- Speak at a steady pace and in simple (non-academic) language.
- Adapt to the person's own pace and preferred communication type and style.
- Explain research terms each time they are used (or use simpler alternatives) and avoid using abbreviations and acronyms.
- Avoid inappropriate exclusion of people, for example because of a diagnosis, deafness or language barrier. Take reasonable steps to be inclusive. For example, offer translators, remote video or telephone conferencing where transport is not available or easily accessible. Avoid limiting your study to an upper age limit without good reason.
- Avoid over-taxing people's memory or communication skills. Always re-cap on previous conversations or interviews each time.

---

3   http://dementiavoices.org.uk/wp-content/uploads/2013/11/DEEP-Guide-Writing-dementia-friendly-information.pdf

- Include enough breaks (e.g. for refreshments, quiet time, toilet and re-focusing) because research involves a lot of concentration.

Obtain feedback

- Ask participants (and if agreed, their families or a trusted person whom they nominate) how they want feedback: at what points and in what ways? This may need to be re-checked.
- Provide a summary of the final report in simple, understandable language. Offer individuals a choice of what type of report they want (e.g. a summary, two sides of key points, or the full report). Confirm this again at the end of their involvement.

Deal with thank-you payments and expenses

- Ensure that these are prompt and require minimal or no form-filling.

Other ways to be involved in research

Not everyone wants to lead a piece of research. Lots of people enjoy being involved in other people's research as a research participant, or as a PPIE ('patient and public involvement and engagement') member or a co-producer. In fact, many people involved in Dementia Enquirers have become more confident as PPIE members or co-producers since their research project. Their expectations are higher and clearer about the kind of role they can expect, and how they can be involved in equal partnership with academic researchers. You can read more about PPIE and co-production and how this sits with our driving seat model in Chapter 8.

Dementia Enquirers has allowed people with dementia to safely navigate and adjust to the research world. There is a power in collective action, with people with dementia joining forces to deliver these projects. The role of peer support and the sharing of responsibilities is something we pick up on in Chapter 6. Dementia Enquirers is based on DEEP values, has the right kind of scaffolding around it, has grown the skills and confidence of people with dementia, and has created a self-belief that 'we are researchers'.

As the Pioneers say: 'We are research gold dust. We can! You can!'

CHAPTER 5

Tackling the Complexities of Research Ethics

I'm just happy if we can influence ethics committees to
see our ability differently. To see our un-vulnerability.
They are forever trying to protect us. (Wendy)

Chapter summary

In this chapter, we explain why ethics are important in research and why some people find current processes inaccessible and unfit for purpose. We also describe how the Pioneers have tried to address the issues head on through the development and application of new Gold Standards.

Background – 'the system'

Ethics in research are undeniably important. In the past, bad things have sometimes been done to vulnerable people because of a lack of scrutiny, and some early research would now certainly be seen as unethical. Research ethics committees (often called RECs) were set up in the late 1960s and early 1970s to stop this type of research from happening today and to safeguard the rights, safety, dignity and wellbeing of research participants.

There are more than 80 NHS RECs across the UK – all come under the Health Research Authority, including the Social Care REC. They consist of up to 15 members, a third of whom are 'lay'. Most universities also have established RECs as part of their internal governance arrangements. All RECs are entirely independent of research sponsors (the organizations responsible for the management and conduct of the research), funders and the researchers themselves. This enables them to put participants at the centre of their review.

RECs review research proposals and give an opinion about whether the research is ethical. They ask researchers to show that their research puts people's wellbeing first, and protects participants from harm. They can also identify risks the researchers haven't thought of, which in turn can help reduce these risks. And they can reassure participants that the researchers have thought about ethics, and the right way to act. They look too at issues such as participant involvement in the research. The diagram below shows the main processes a research team often has to go through before it can start any research:

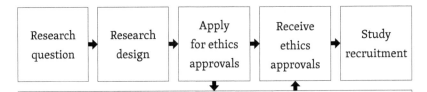

- Justify the research focus
- Explain the methodology and research process
- Explore ethical considerations and how you will minimize any negative impact
- Prepare research materials, e.g. information sheets and consent forms
- Have work reviewed by research ethics committee

Courtesy of Dr Rosie Ashworth

ETHICS PROCESS

Why were ethics systems an issue for Dementia Enquirers?

'Being ethical' in research is really just about being honest, respectful and appropriately careful towards anyone involved in your project. An ethical research project is one that:

- is honest and clear
- is respectful of everyone taking part
- looks after the health and wellbeing of people taking part
- has a clear plan to complete the research
- has a clear purpose/reason to be done.

Being ethical, in the broadest sense of the word, was a position that people with dementia held as the cornerstone of Dementia Enquirers. Many people had experienced being participants in research that did not follow the principles listed above.

Although no one would want their research to be *unethical*, not all projects are required to go through an ethics approval process – for example, if you're finding people through contacts, adverts, social media and so on, or if the research is a stand-alone evaluation of a service (including a survey). But the criteria in themselves can be hard to establish for a specific project.

For academic researchers, thinking about ethics in research results in a direct pathway to research ethics committees, where researchers spell out their planned practices, which are then judged to be ethical or not. However, when approval is required, the process can often feel very daunting and inaccessible (not only to people who aren't familiar with it, but also to people who are!). It is often hard to know which REC(s) you would go to, what kind of approval you need, and what happens during the approval process.

This is even more the case for people with dementia who want to lead their own research – they are often thought incapable of even consenting to research, let alone leading it. And this is contrary to how people with dementia want to do research:

> We want to encourage more people with the lived experience of dementia to do their own research on what matters to them. (Dory)

> We want our research to include, not exclude – and to assume that people with dementia have capacity as the starting point. (Ron)

> People with dementia have a sense of urgency for action and change – so we don't want processes that slow us down. (Agnes)

We quickly discovered that if people with dementia want to design and lead their own research, they have no direct route to any organized REC. They will effectively need to partner with an organization that does research (such as a university or hospital) as these will either have a REC, or access to one.

Also, there are seemingly different (and inconsistent) processes between many of the different RECs (in particular, universities). The systems can often feel complicated, jargon-ridden, time-consuming, resource-draining and de-skilling. And not only that: some of the processes themselves seem actually *un*ethical – or at least not central to what is or should be ethical about a project!

But there is a Catch-22. If REC approval is not asked for and gained, the work may not be taken seriously by other researchers, and it may not be publishable in reputable academic journals. This matters, because publishing research in peer-reviewed journals is the best way to have research read by an international academic and clinical audience, and thus to have the greatest impact. In some ways, this is a good thing, as it means you can't do whatever you want and then try to publish it (without considering ethics or the participants' wellbeing). But the current options are too restrictive, and they mean that it is much harder for research by people with dementia to be taken seriously and to reach the right audiences. This is contrary to what people with dementia want:

> We want our findings to be taken seriously by other researchers, and to publish in academic ('peer-reviewed') journals. But can we do that if we don't get REC approval? (Mhari)

Dementia Enquirers Ethics Seminar

The research methods pack (described in Chapter 2), which was completed and published in 2019 (and revised 2023) (Innovations in Dementia, 2023a), already highlighted some of these issues, and suggested questions that researchers need to ask themselves. However, we started to think we should proceed with creating our own resource about ethics. In order to progress our thinking and practice we held a seminar in London in February 2020. This involved the Pioneers, and a number of invited academics and ethicists. The former were able to highlight their frustrations about, and the perceived limitations of, the current system, while the latter provided some much-needed grounding in the law and protocols involved in ethical approval needed for research. Everyone agreed that the system needed reforming.

The event generated wide-ranging discussions about what needed to be done next and identified key issues:

- how to recognize and minimize differences in power
- how to demonstrate respect and consideration to all involved
- how to protect participants from harm (physical and emotional) – and minimize any potential risks
- how to ensure that consent is supported and informed
- confidentiality/anonymity
- acknowledgement
- accessible information
- ethics approval
- how to make sure the reviewers and the researchers understand dementia.

It was felt that the current culture of RECs is inaccessible (even for junior researchers) – one participant described them as 'the last bastion of paternalism'. There was consensus that a different or separate process is really important to challenge the orthodoxy. There was even discussion about the idea and feasibility of a new ethics panel. Do read Wendy Mitchell's blog[1] about this event, and listen to George's Dementia Diary.[2]

Creating the new Gold Standards

The discussions at the seminar in February 2000 formed the basis for a major new stream of work – the development of *The DEEP-Ethics Gold Standards* (later revised to *The Dementia Enquirers Gold Standards for Ethical Research*) (Innovations in Dementia, 2023b). This work highlighted that ethics affect every aspect of research – it's so much more than just getting a proposal through a committee. We have shown how, once we make the language, systems and concepts more accessible, people with dementia (and many others) *can* engage with ethics processes with enthusiasm. Not only that, but involving people with dementia in ethics processes can actually broaden the scope and impact of research.

---

1   https://whichmeamitoday.wordpress.com/2020/02/13/another-trundle-back-down-to-london

2   https://dementiadiaries.org/entry/13749/george-reports-from-a-recent-meeting-of-dementia-enquirers

The Standards are an attempt to pilot a new system which:

- is more flexible, and can take a considered approach to some of the grey areas
- respects the sense of urgency of the need for action and change that people with dementia feel
- incorporates support for people to make their own decisions
- is realistic about how we think about risk
- starts from the assumption that being diagnosed with dementia does not mean you necessarily lack capacity; wants to include (not exclude), and assumes that people have got capacity to be involved (unless it is shown that they don't) – in line with the Mental Capacity Act (and similar legislation in Scotland and Northern Ireland)
- focuses less on *why* the project is being done, and more on whether *how* it is being done is ethical
- respects the importance of equality and diversity issues, and the requirements of the Equality Act for 'reasonable adjustments'.

With this mandate from the seminar, we co-produced the Standards through the spring and early summer of 2020 (during the first lockdown), with a lot of help from our advisors and allies. We also drew on a number of phone interviews which were carried out with experts in various fields. For a full list of those who helped us, please see Acknowledgments.

We also drew on a range of important guidelines – from the Health Research Authority (n.d.), the British Society of Gerontology (2012), the British Psychological Society (2021), the Economic and Social Research Council (2022), and the Wellcome Trust (2014). The guidelines drawn up by the Scottish Dementia Working Group (2013) are of particular significance.

The Gold Standards are based on six principles which have been identified by people with dementia who are involved in research (or want to be involved).

The aim of the Gold Standards checklist that follows is not only to make sure that the research is being carried out legally, and in line with ethical requirements, but also to provide reassurance that the project has been carefully thought through. Those who need to know this include:

- people with dementia who are involved (and their families/advocates)
- any academic partners
- policymakers, organizations and local authorities that may consider changes to policies or practices as a result of the research
- any organizations that might be involved (e.g. in providing access as a research 'site')
- journals which may consider publishing findings.

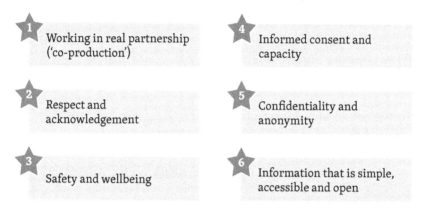

THE GOLD STANDARD'S SIX PRINCIPLES

Ethics in our own application processes

At the time of the applications for cohort 1 (summer 2019) we had not drawn up the Gold Standards. However, we did require applicants to consider ethics issues. Following on from the ethics seminar (see above) we agreed to pilot the Standards on the next round of applications we received from groups in the DEEP (Dementia Engagement and Empowerment Project) network for funding (cohort 2: summer 2020).

Prior to actually assessing cohort-2 applications, the Pioneers practised using the Standards with support from Dr Lucy Series, a mental health law expert from the University of Cardiff. They used an agreed checklist of nine main points (see below) on a 'dummy' proposal. They then reviewed the actual applications and made recommendations. You can watch a film of the Pioneers working through this process.[3]

---

3   www.youtube.com/watch?v=Xe07OUuWt1Q&feature=youtu.be

Cohort 2 checklist – ethics issues

☐ 1. Is it clear what is planned?
☐ 2. Have they thought about consent processes?
☐ 3. Have they mentioned a written information sheet?
☐ 4. Would it be possible to easily recognize the participants?
☐ 5. Will they discuss this with people?
☐ 6. Will they anonymize people if necessary?
☐ 7. Will they feed back to participants at the end of the project?
☐ 8. How accessible will the project materials be? (May be a worry if the application itself isn't very accessible.)
☐ 9. Does the project feel 'invasive'? If so, check more fully in the Ethics Gold Standards.

In the actual application process, a small number of projects were rejected because they did not meet the Standards. The checklist gave the Pioneers confidence and 'permission' to do so.

The Pioneers gave very positive feedback on the process of using the Standards:

I used the six principles as a guide the whole time. I felt that the DEEP ones gave a really good basis to make decisions on. I did not have to feel in a quandary at all because the ethics were quite clearly stated. These are hugely helpful. (Irene)

I felt it was good to learn how to use the tool – and in using it, it got your head to think [about] the principles... The principles have helped simplify what could be a very complex area for me. (Agnes)

I found it made it clearer and simpler to work out the ethics... I'm not very good at putting across the words, I forget all the words. (Dory)

Yes...that's total control. I love it...it made me look a lot deeper into the proposals, and think a lot more about them. (Steve)

Ethics in the individual DEEP projects

Ethics can sound mysterious and worrying. But 'being ethical' in research is really just about being honest, respectful and appropriately careful towards anyone involved in your research project.

In the case of most of the Dementia Enquirers projects, research ethics committees were not open to DEEP groups, or were not a necessary part of establishing an ethical approach. Nevertheless, being ethical was still a principle that people with dementia wanted to achieve. Ethics processes were not always accessible or understandable to people with dementia. But the principle of 'being ethical' was.

In cohort 1, the York Minds and Voices group carried out a project on the pros and cons, and the particular needs, of people with dementia who live alone and those who live with a care partner. They originally planned to obtain ethical approval from the University of Hull. In their report,[4] they give us a flavour of how off-putting these processes are for people with dementia:

> The documents that came through relating to gaining ethical approval for a piece of research were wholly inappropriate in terms of the detail requested. It was set up to have a University academic with a University email as principal investigator which immediately takes away the ownership of the project from members of Minds and Voices – defeating the object of people with dementia being in the driving seat... The approval process was too big and daunting for us given the time available. It really did not fit who we are and was geared up for people already working as researchers within the university.

Also in cohort 1, Our Voice Matters (Hartlepool) looked at the impact of community-based groups on people with dementia. In their report,[5] they describe a similar experience:

> From conducting this research, one of the main things we have learnt is that you have to be very careful when involving other organizations. When we started off, one of the areas we wanted to research was a group

---

4   https://dementiaenquirers.org.uk/wp-content/uploads/2021/05/minds-and-voices-in-york_report.pdf

5   https://dementiaenquirers.org.uk/wp-content/uploads/2021/05/our-voice-matters-in-hartlepool_report.pdf

run through the NHS. For us to be able to do this we would have been required to go through their ethics board and have all of the research signed off and approved. Once learning this information, we decided to rethink the direction of the research, to something that was more generalized and that didn't need to go through another company's ethics board.

Some projects which did go through the REC process experienced delays that were disproportionate to the total length of the project (one year). For example, Ashford Phoenix and the Canterbury Forget-Me-Nots research group both used up six months to get their REC approval. The Up and Go group (Leeds) had to leave this process to the academics because of pressure of time. This went against their collaborative approach but was a pragmatic decision based on the complexity of the process.

Engaging with academics on ethics issues

With the help of Dr Lucy Series, we made contact with Professor Michael Dunn (Associate Professor at Oxford University), whose work revolves around research ethics. In September 2020, he kindly agreed to be interviewed by two of our Pioneers – George Rook and Mhari McLintock – about some of the myths that surround ethics and dementia. George and Mhari drew up a list of the 'myths' that they wanted to discuss with Professor Dunn:

- All people with dementia lack capacity and require special research processes.
- Other people can consent to participation on behalf of a person with dementia.
- Only doctors can assess capacity.
- People with dementia cannot conduct research.
- People with dementia cannot understand ethics or come to considered judgements about capacity, consent and the risk of harm.
- People with dementia doing research have nothing to teach academics.
- Mainstream research and research governance have no need to adapt, to include people with dementia.

- If we involved people with dementia we would have to redesign the questions and that would invalidate the research.
- It's too difficult to find people with dementia.
- It's too time-consuming to involve people with dementia.
- You have to have full academic training and experience to understand and apply ethics to research.
- Ethics is a highly specialized discipline. Lay people, especially those with dementia, cannot possibly understand or use ethics principles.
- People with dementia cannot remember things, so how can they answer questions?
- People with dementia cannot understand research questions, and we cannot rely on their answers.

This resulted in a fascinating discussion which was filmed.[6] It was not just the content but also the process which was ground-breaking. It is refreshing to see two people living with dementia interviewing an academic expert with such confidence.

Dr Chiara De Poli is a research officer at the London School of Economics and Political Science (LSE). One of her research interests is in research ethics and in finding solutions to ethics issues like the ones we have been discussing. She has worked with colleagues and researchers and identified some ideas that could improve how research ethics committees think about and deal with collaborative research involving people living with dementia. In 2022, Chiara was awarded an NIHR (National Institute for Health and Care Research) grant to expand on this by including the perspectives of organizations working with vulnerable groups, vulnerable individuals themselves, research funding bodies, university RECs and the Health Research Authority. This exploratory work will be used to prepare a research proposal aiming to facilitate real change in the English ethics system for social care research, which ultimately should widen inclusion and participation in research. Chiara is using the *Dementia Enquirers Gold Standards for Ethical Research* as an example of 'spontaneous', bottom-up initiatives which are trialling solutions to address the specificities of doing participatory research with vulnerable populations.

Dr Rosie Ashworth, an advisor to Dementia Enquirers, led a co-

---

6   www.youtube.com/watch?v=wdWSn-1glko&feature=youtu.be

produced scoping review to explore the inclusion of people with dementia in the ethical review process. Dr Ashworth has been working on a scoping review of reports of people with dementia (or with lived experience of health conditions) being included in the ethics process. She narrowed down 70 titles for an abstract screening, and Pioneers and other advisors volunteered to be reviewers of the abstracts. Rosie did a great job of making the whole process as accessible as possible! Her findings were as follows:

- People with dementia have an important and unique perspective on research about dementia.
- No published examples were found. However, there were a few (unpublished) cases of people with lived experience running an ethics committee. Although they were not people specifically with dementia, it shows that this is possible.
- More research is needed to explore how research ethics committees make decisions about dementia research.
- Researchers should be clearer and more detailed about their ethics approvals, and about whether people with dementia were involved in the review.

At the time of writing this book, the scoping review is waiting for acceptance for publication.

In 2022, academics at the University of Stirling committed to integrating the Standards into their international online MSc in Dementia Studies course, the largest in the world. The Pioneers started the process by delivering an online session explaining their perspectives on research ethics and processes. They then responded to issues raised on the 'discussion board', as the students began to integrate the Standards into their project assignments. Finally, the students fed back to the Pioneers on how the Standards had influenced their thinking. This is summed up here by the course leaders:

This session was really useful for students and staff – thank you very much Pioneers. Your guidance on ethical dementia research is a fantastic tool and will be incredibly helpful for anyone designing a research project and thinking about ethics approval. (Dr Richard Ward, Senior Lecturer in Dementia Studies, Faculty of Social Sciences)

It's definitely inspired [our students] as they continue with their studies... I think you'll have encouraged them all to think about their future professional work in much more inclusive and participatory ways. (Dr Grant Gibson, Lecturer in Dementia Studies, Faculty of Social Sciences)

The World Health Organization (WHO)

One of the Pioneers, who is involved with the WHO's Global Dementia Observatory Knowledge Exchange (GDO KE) platform, arranged for the Gold Standards to be included on this platform.[7] The GDO KE platform enhances countries' and communities' response to dementia by sharing resources at no cost, facilitating mutual learning and promoting the exchange of knowledge. It contains key resources to support the implementation of the *Global Action Plan on the Public Health Response to Dementia 2017–2025* (World Health Organization, 2017) and its seven action areas.

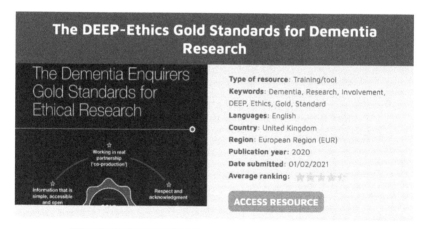

SCREENSHOT FROM THE GLOBAL DEMENTIA OBSERVATORY
KNOWLEDGE EXCHANGE PLATFORM

What next?

Our work on ethics has shown that once we make the language, systems and concepts more accessible, people with dementia (and many others!)

---

7   https://globaldementia.org/en/resource/the-deep-ethics-gold-standards-for-dementia-research

can engage with them with enthusiasm. Not only that, but they broaden the scope of research, and refine the practicalities.

In the final year of the programme (2022–23) we were engaged in active discussion with the Health Research Authority (HRA). As part of their 'Think Ethics' pilot, two of the Pioneers were invited to observe a REC session and they reported back on their reflections. We are hopeful that their observations will make a difference.

In the light of our work, we hope that RECs will encourage researchers to be guided by the Gold Standards as they start to draft their proposals; before submitting to a funder; before submitting to a REC; and throughout the whole process of fieldwork, analysis, reporting and dissemination.

RECs also have a key role to play in:

- accepting that people with dementia can be in the driving seat of research
- making their own processes and language simpler and more accessible (though still in line with regulatory requirements)
- expecting that research involving, or carried out by, people with dementia uses simpler and more accessible methods – and that these are not unethical
- accepting that if a project follows the Gold Standards, this is evidence that it is ethical (though this will not always mean that REC approval is not needed).

We believe that the outcomes from these actions will be significant because:

- standards of research involving people with dementia will rise, and the skills and confidence of researchers to involve people with dementia will increase
- research will reflect much more closely the priorities of people with dementia (e.g. in relation to research design and conduct) and make the most of all they can contribute
- research teams will have more thorough discussions about research ethics when working co-productively
- many more people with dementia will feel confident to be involved in research, in whatever capacity.

We also hope that:

- funders may suggest (or require) that projects they fund follow the Gold Standards
- more researchers may voluntarily decide to use the Gold Standards
- peer-reviewed journals will accept the Gold Standards as evidence that a project is ethical.

CHAPTER 6

What Does This All Mean for DEEP Group Members and Facilitators?

*We're all unique and wonderful – but
together we're a masterpiece. (Dory)*

Chapter summary

Dementia Enquirers has been about increasing the skills and knowledge of people with dementia to lead their own research, while also trying to make the world of research more accessible and welcoming to them.

Throughout the programme, we have invited feedback and reflection from all those involved, and in particular from the people with dementia. This includes, of course, both the Pioneers, who have shaped the programme alongside us, and the members of the many DEEP (Dementia Engagement and Empowerment Project) groups who have carried out their own research. In many cases, we have filmed the discussions. A number of the final project reports also include fascinating reflections about what the work actually meant for the people with dementia who led it.

Drawing on this evidence, we look in this chapter at the demands on group members and facilitators, the different roles they took on, and also some of the tensions and different expectations that arose within the groups. While the feedback from all involved has overall been very positive, it is fair to say that each group has taken on the challenge of being 'in the driving seat' in its own way. Nevertheless, the outcomes for the people with dementia have, by their own testimony, been substantial – and in some cases, life-changing.

Getting started

Groups used their modest grants in different ways. Some used them to pay the facilitator and/or the group members for their time. Some of their money was allocated to practical costs such as venues and transport – though these budget headings were often under-used when the Covid-19 lockdowns came into force. A few groups allocated funds to specific project requirements such as a trip out or a piece of equipment.

Deciding on a research question is the exciting bit! The processes we have tested out show that people with dementia know the research questions that they want answering. Their lived experience puts them in a very good position to say what dementia research should be about. It turns out that their research questions are very different from other people's. The issues that they spend time talking about in their DEEP groups were perfect for researching further. The 26 Dementia Enquirers projects were all based on topics that people found important, reflecting day-to-day struggles and social barriers, as well as hopes. They looked at things like living alone, using Alexa, the diagnosis experience, transport, music-making and discrimination.

Learning new skills

People with dementia have learned lots of new things by running their own research projects:

- looking at other people's research about their topic
- creating a questionnaire
- interviewing other people with dementia
- making a film
- thinking about what their results mean
- writing research reports and articles
- making suggestions about what needs to change because of what they have found out.

People with dementia say that running a research project is hard work but enjoyable and stimulating, and massively builds confidence. By working as a team, people with dementia have been able to play to their strengths. People could do the job they had an interest or skills in. This is exactly how research teams work in universities!

Negotiating roles and levels of control

In most of the Dementia Enquirers projects, the people with dementia needed – and drew on – support from others. There was no expectation that they should do everything themselves. Most, but not all, of the groups were supported in their research by their usual facilitator. These facilitators were rarely employed by the group itself – they could be employed by a charity, by a university or by a Health Trust. Sometimes the facilitator was a carer or former carer. In a few cases, they were a person living with dementia themselves. In addition, there were often others involved – volunteers, students or local researchers. So the groups came with a wide range of knowledge about doing research: some were very experienced, while others had done none at all. This point also affected the kind of resources and networks they were able to tap into on behalf of the group.

DEEP group facilitators proved to be a good source of practical support. In the projects, they often:

- made appointments
- put a questionnaire on the internet
- wrote up notes from interviews and team discussions
- organized team meetings for the researchers.

In short, they acted as general assistants to the researchers with dementia. Of course, many people with dementia also took on some of the jobs above. It all depended on people's skills and interests. The most important point is that people with dementia continued to *lead and control* the research.

In terms of the level of control of individual members, it is perhaps unsurprising that these were very varied. Some inevitably had more skills, experience, time, confidence, energy or enthusiasm than others. Some were at an early stage of dementia, others a bit further down the road. The trick was to identify these aspects at the start so that each person could contribute in the way they wanted and felt able to.

Helping people with dementia to be in the driving seat is easier said than done. What does it mean exactly? On occasion, there were tensions because of a mismatch of expectations. In one group, for example, it was reported that one member felt that she could and should be in a real leadership role (with assistance where needed), while other team members, and the group facilitators, felt that the main fieldwork and data collection should be done by a professional, with the project team as advisors. This misunderstanding led to some changes in the support arrangements mid-project. The report[1] concludes:

> It is fair to say that this caused a certain amount of difficulty for the project – which, with hindsight, could have been reduced by very early agreement about expectations, skillsets and roles.

The facilitator of this group commented in the report:

> While facilitators have made opportunities available to people with dementia to take on project team work – chairing meetings, designing logos, helping design feedback forms and writing the report – most project team members were clear they did not want these roles and identified some of them as overwhelming. By answering their questions, project members wanted to learn about Alexa and help others to do the same. They did this as experts by experience, using their ability to learn and teach at the same time, helping to produce the valuable information that can now be shared and evaluated. This approach comes naturally to group members, as they have been using it for many years when helping deliver dementia training. This is our take on being 'in the driving seat'.

The 26 projects have shown us that there are many ways to negotiate their own way of working. For example, the Shrewsbury Riversiders and York Minds and Voices groups worked together on a project about the interaction between DEEP groups and Admiral Nurses.[2] Their experience was that:

> The focus required has to be applied, usually by one person, after getting consent and support from others. Everyone has different experiences and skills. The trick is probably to find an issue to research, which encompasses a good number of group members' interests and experiences... Who does the work? Who has the skills? What skills do we

1   https://dementiaenquirers.org.uk/wp-content/uploads/2021/05/educate-in-stock port_report.pdf
2   https://dementiaenquirers.org.uk/wp-content/uploads/2021/05/riversiders-in-shrewsbury-with-minds-and-voices-york_report.pdf

need? What equipment do we need, and can we use it? These dictate who does the work.

The Forget-me-nots group looked at how Covid-19 has affected people with dementia in Kent, in relation to technology, relationships, coping and physical and mental health. Their project was led by a working party comprising people with dementia, students and volunteers. They described their process of negotiation in their report:[3]

> We have learned some valuable lessons about Enquiry writing in general that made our project both functional and unique. Firstly, communication played an important part in our project, with the working party and students/volunteers constantly contacting one another, allowing the project to run very smoothly. Part of this communication was our ability to disagree with each other, yet still come to constructive conclusions that allowed us to move forward with the Enquiry in a way that was helpful and productive.

Few, if any, of the groups could have carried out their enquiries without the support of the facilitators – most (though not all) of whom were *not* living with dementia. However, the sharing of power and the negotiating of roles in order to come as close as possible to the 'driving seat' aspiration was not an easy ask. Groups took a range of approaches and it is fair to say that some found it much more difficult than others. However, there is very rich learning to be had from their honest feedback.

A large part of the facilitator role has been making the *processes* as accessible as possible, and so enabling each project member to play the role they wanted to play. Paula Brown, facilitator of the Scottish Dementia Alumni, said:

> My facilitation role has been about removing barriers and easing access – the ideas, development and testing of the resource has been entirely attributable to the group members and their collaborators.

In the York Minds and Voices project, for example, Damian worked

---

3   https://dementiaenquirers.org.uk/wp-content/uploads/2021/10/10106a_de-report-forget-me-nots-october-2021.pdf

with group member Brian on the literature reviews, as highlighted in a short film.[4]

Likewise, in the report[5] from the Up and Go Leeds group:

> When we met at the Playhouse for the data analysis there were certain things that I didn't take in, and Nicky and Elizabeth both explained it to me. So it took a bit of time, but it did go in. Even then, I didn't feel on a lower level, it's just it was something that I didn't understand. So I felt both were approachable in how they said things and it helped me to have a better understanding.

Other group members confirmed the importance of this patient (and time-consuming) approach:

> Meeting every fortnight was good and sending us all notes of what had happened so we could read it at home and digest it, that was helpful.

> It was stepped, so every question was 'What do you think about the wording for this?' and if you wanted to change something, it was changed. It was done in stages.

In the THRED project, Pat and Louise (former carers, not living with dementia) supported the organization, management, marketing, delivery and analysis of the project. However, Tommy and Paul (both living with dementia) carried out all the fieldwork, applied their own creative methods and also wrote the report:[6]

> Tommy and Paul developed relevant questions for surveys; met and engaged with DEEP groups and others; [and] interviewed and filmed discussions they had with different groups across the UK. Additionally, they followed up their research to highlight emerging issues through THRED's weekly Twitter chat. It became clear early on in the project that Tommy and Paul had the credibility with their peers to open up

---

4   www.youtube.com/watch?v=oUgTpADlauY&t=10s
5   https://dementiaenquirers.org.uk/wp-content/uploads/2022/11/up-and-go-leeds-oct-2022-report.pdf
6   https://dementiaenquirers.org.uk/wp-content/uploads/2021/05/thred-in-liverpool_report.pdf

trusted conversations and understanding of the transport issues raised, which provided a platform to dig deeper as a researcher.

From all the feedback and reflections we have come up with a number of key learning points. Facilitators can and should have confidence in the potential of people with dementia to do research. They can enable people with dementia to be in the driving seat by helping them to:

- write proposals and funding bids
- access useful partners (e.g. local academics or students)
- make processes and information as accessible and personalized as possible
- carry out some or all of the background administrative tasks
- identify what skills they have, and what roles each person wants to take on.

However, all this can and does take skill and confidence on the part of the facilitators. Some will already have academic experience – and for them, letting go of control will not be easy. Others will have little or no academic experience – and, for them, even the words 'university' and 'research' may be quite scary. The latter will need a lot of support and probably an academic partner who is willing to share the load and make it more accessible. The resources produced during the programme, and in particular *How To Do a Research Project* (Innovations in Dementia, 2023a) should be very helpful.

Group culture

One of the key factors is the existing culture of the group – and the philosophy, confidence, attitude and skills of the facilitator. With our focus on the people with dementia themselves, this is something to which, with hindsight, we did not give enough attention. As the EDU-CATE report highlights (see Case Study 2, Appendix 2), in some groups members felt that they could and should be in a real leadership role (with assistance where needed). In other groups, facilitators (and perhaps the members too) felt that the main fieldwork and data collection should be done by a professional, with the members as advisors. If the facilitator is already used to *enabling* rather than *running* the group, the former (the ultimate 'in the driving seat' approach) will come much more naturally. And even if facilitators have little research confidence themselves, they will treat the project as a joint adventure in which they and the members learn and develop skills alongside each other.

What all this shows perhaps is the absolute importance of clarity about roles and expectations right from the very start of the project – though with enough flexibility built in to enable all to develop, experiment and flourish.

Other issues experienced

Time was another key factor, as Nicky Taylor, facilitator of Up and Go in Leeds, explains:

> It has been a significant piece of work which has taken well over the number of days I was allocated for it. I think that is due to my ways of working but also demonstrates the commitment needed when engaging people meaningfully in co-production – I am yet to crack the balance of this, despite numerous similar projects.

Some facilitators have only a few paid hours a week (or even a month) to help run their group – extra projects such as these demand a lot of extra input and should be funded accordingly. But even if the funding for extra time is available, the facilitator may not *have* extra time to commit.

Project teams were given a year to complete their work. In a number of cases, they did say that they felt rushed. Some groups found it difficult to fit in the extra meetings required – one even found they had to meet every week at times. Time lags associated with ethics approvals, survey responses and so on also affected their timetables. These issues could add unwelcome pressure to those involved.

Working together across more than one group was also a challenge. As the Shrewsbury Riversiders explained:

> If they are close, and you can meet, it will of course be relatively easy. At a distance, as we were, we managed to meet in person at a halfway place, Stockport... I found on the web, and hired, a community space close to the station, and ordered in lunch from a recommended nearby shop. Those who attended did a really good job of challenging what I

thought were already pretty watertight survey questions! So I changed quite a lot of detail afterwards. It was also just a good day of chat and discussion. That was a powerful spin off, and without Covid we would have met again.

Another barrier to overcome was the difference in ability of group members. In their report on the effect of class, ethnicity and intellect on the dementia pathway, the Beth Johnson Foundation[7] group explain:

As in any type of groups, there are members who are able to express themselves more readily than others. In the development of this project, as members were in the driving seat, they have facilitated those members who were not as confident, ensuring that all members had an equal share of the participation of the project.

The global pandemic undoubtedly had an impact on the programme and on the individual projects too. Many had to revise their aspirations and methodologies. However, we were impressed with how practicable it was to do this. The report[8] by the Shrewsbury Riversiders and York Minds and Voices describes some adjustments that they had to make in their joint project:

Several Riversiders have highly relevant and useful skills, although due to lockdown it was almost impossible to work together on the project. George led it, but discussed ideas and approaches with Riversiders via Zoom. While planning it, George worked out research approaches and questions and agreed these in outline with Damian [the facilitator of York Minds and Voices]. Then drafts were given to Riversiders, and three people responded with detailed suggestions. Two Riversiders (plus one spouse) met two York Minds and Voices members plus Damian in Stockport for half a day, lunch included, to test the surveys for wording, clarity and answerability. Changes were subsequently made by George… The questions were tested out by George visiting a Birmingham CPD (Continuing Professional Development) Admiral Nurse group.

---

7   https://dementiaenquirers.org.uk/wp-content/uploads/2021/05/beth_johnson_foundation_in_stoke-on-trent_report.pdf

8   https://dementiaenquirers.org.uk/wp-content/uploads/2021/05/riversiders-in-shrewsbury-with-minds-and-voices-york_report.pdf

But having to adapt to the lockdown was not necessarily a bad thing. As the Beth Johnson Foundation report explains, having to find new ways of working due to Covid-19 actually increased their self-confidence in using different methods. And groups took pride in the fact that, by continuing the programme in spite of the pandemic, they had shown university teams what was possible!

Another barrier was the ethics processes, which have already been discussed in an earlier chapter.

What about carers?

This programme of work was very much about the voice of people with dementia themselves – not that of carers, supporters or professionals. But it is not the case that carers have played no part in it. One group, for example (THRED) is facilitated/supported by former carers. Also, some individual Dementia Enquirers have had substantial support from their care partner, for example in bringing them to meetings or even residential gatherings, and helping them to interpret information.

We hope carers will not feel excluded by this approach, but will recognize the importance of enabling people with dementia to have their voices heard directly. This shouldn't set up a false conflict. Were this the case, it would be an unhelpful distraction.

Outcomes for groups and individuals with dementia

From the feedback received, and from the reports themselves, we have identified the following five key outcomes for people with dementia:

- pride in making an impact
- growth in confidence, self-worth and meaning
- playing to strengths and developing skills
- influencing academics and the research agenda
- inclusion, belonging and teamwork.

1. Pride in making an impact

Undoubtedly, one of the main motivations for people with dementia to be involved in research is the hope that they can make an impact, if only on future generations. Many spoke of their 'passion to change things'. The DEEP groups were determined to ensure this was the case:

> These reports are going to be an asset, coming out of Covid. They won't sit on the shelf... So much effort's gone in to them, I'm damned if we'll let it! (Agnes, DEEP researcher)

Two of the groups were very proud that they were launching their reports in Dementia Action Week.

Just having their own voices heard and listened to felt like a big achievement:

> One member said how good it felt to be listened to and know that what he was saying was being used in a purposeful manner in the project... (Beth Johnson Foundation group member)

> There's a massive shift now towards the academics hearing our voices... and I'm glad about that. (Paul, DEEP researcher)

Groups were particularly encouraged when they could see some clear impact from their work. The Shrewsbury Riversiders made sure that they had the ownership of a key stakeholder right from the start:

> Dementia UK were involved...at early stages and for consultation at various stages, to ensure they felt involved, and would therefore be committed to action following the project's findings... The second draft was shared with Dementia UK. A month later, Damian [facilitator] and I [George] met online with the Dementia UK Clinical Director and one of the LEAP[9] facilitators/consultant Admiral Nurses. We agreed several actions that both sides committed to, and were incorporated onto the draft.

All this is not to say that leading a research project, however small, is easy. But the overcoming of fears, and the hard work put in, make the pride even stronger:

---

9   LEAP stands for Lived Experience Advisory Panel.

I'm just glad we achieved it. At first I was worried that we might not, but as we went on I thought, 'Yes, we can do it', and we did it!

All the hard work we did, it's coming into fruition in the very near future. We did this!

Way back when we started it, it did feel like we had a mountain to climb!

2. Growth in confidence, self-worth and meaning

Being in the driving seat of research doesn't mean that you have to do everything yourself. Teamwork and support can really help. But controlling the research and leading the way give people with dementia a huge boost in confidence. This was often described as very empowering – even transformative:

I thought it was wonderful. My name was mentioned – and other people's – and it was great. I kept reading it and reading it! In fact, my friend is coming round later and I'm going to show it to her. (Joan)

I felt very uneasy the first few meetings because I was stepping out of my comfort zone. But as the process went on, as we attended more meetings, I began to feel more confident in myself. And I enjoyed it.

For some, it was an important stage in acknowledging, and moving on from, their diagnosis. They spoke of the 'fight' they had had to be accepted, to 'prove myself', to 'blow away prejudices'. They explained that joining this programme was 'liberating', 'vindicating' and 'confirming'. The projects clearly had a real impact on self-belief and confidence, changing the way in which people with dementia saw themselves:

I am a researcher...who has dementia. (Martin)

The research side of it was absolutely fascinating... I read the full report and it was amazing, well put together, easy to read...and I was very, very proud of the final report – brilliant. (Steve)

It's changed my life. I can still be useful. (Dory)

We ended up with a 42-page report about how we benefitted from it [making-music] and how it made us feel. And we've also got a 25-minute video...which shows the whole process from being brand-new and raw, to lovely, soft tender fingers, to blistered fingers, as it were... We're very proud of it, and...we intend to share that with as many people as we can. (Chris)

I think it's achieved so much in changing perspective, busting through mythologies, prejudices, assumptions. (Daithi)

3. Playing to strengths and developing skills

People living with dementia generally have many decades of life experience behind them – experience in work, in relationships and as citizens. One of the aims of the programme was to find out the extent to which those skills could be unearthed, polished up and celebrated. This was about not only research skills, but also skills in teamwork, time-keeping, talking and listening, writing, analysis and creativity. Those who had specific skills were able to demonstrate them to, and share them with, others in their projects:

> When I got my diagnosis, I initially was positive, and then I allowed the rest of the world, really, to disable me. But through the support of the Pioneers I learned that I could still really well look at a project, or look at a piece of work, or listen to somebody's take on a project. It's been the thing that has given me my persona back. (Irene)

We can shed our dementia skins – come out.

Pat, one of the facilitators of the THRED project, describes in their report how group members Tommy and Paul learned new skills in recording, interviewing and analysing the outcomes of the project. Tommy used his professional reporting skills and, with Paul, drew conclusions on the information and feedback people living with dementia had given, to highlight issues raised and propose potential solutions. But they also drew on their life skills and personalities to enhance their work:

> The additional element that really helped this project was the creative and diverse approach that both Tommy and Paul used when engaging

their peers. They engaged creatively with different groups using original music, humour and role play to gather feedback, views and information on transport issues.

Their enthusiasm was actually a revelation to Pat:

> [They] just completely threw themselves into it. It's something they've felt quite passionate [about] for a long time. This opened up the rest of the country to them... I think they've done a superb job.

Paula, facilitator of the Scottish Dementia Alumni, had a similar reflection about their project producing an educational game for children:

> It was absolutely wonderful to see all of the group members finding creative ways to work on an equal level alongside teachers, children, neuroscientists and each other, and creating ways to scale this work beyond its current capabilities.

Other group members explained the confidence they had got from learning new skills, for example how to work a camera, carry out interviews or set up an online survey. As George explained:

> We learned a huge amount, and it's the learning from doing rather than doing what you're told to do... I think it's important for groups to actually work things out as much as they can for themselves.

In the York Minds and Voices project, Damian, the group facilitator, helped Brian, a group member, to develop skills in literature review. Together they looked over about ten abstracts from Google Scholar. Damian comments that it was only after he simplified the 'impenetrable' abstracts that Brian could give his feedback. Brian was also delighted to find that he *could* make useful comments on research findings as long as they were made accessible to him:

> I'm not intelligent but I know what's what and what's not. All these names they've come up for things is a load of crap... Just make sure that everything written down is clear enough for everyone to read.

Developing new skills (or brushing up on old ones) brought group members a lot of joy:

> I'm blowing my own trumpet, but I just happen to have the skills and work experience to do all this stuff. It's sort of bread and butter to me, and I enjoyed reactivating my brain... (George)

> We actually had a brilliant time doing this. It allowed us all to use our individual talents... Various people took on various roles – it enabled everybody to be involved in it... We came up with some fascinating outcomes. (Wendy)

Many also realized that they still had 'a lifetime of skills and knowledge' that could be put to good use in their project – not necessarily research skills, but transferable skills such as time management, writing, listening or even illustrating.

4. Influencing academics and the research agenda

Those involved in the programme were always clear that they were not trying in any way to be, or to replace, academics. It was often very helpful to involve other academic researchers, given their knowledge and experience of carrying out good quality research. They could also facilitate access to ethics systems, academic journals, data analysis skills and so on. Again, the key was to make sure they knew how to work *alongside* people with dementia, and not take over.

Leading their own research gave some of the DEEP groups new respect for the complexity of research and a better understanding of its many components. As Wendy put it:

> We're not naive enough to think that we could have started with nothing. We've got to have help.

However, they were also clear that they could offer something *different and complementary*. Mark, one of the facilitators, reflected on this at a meeting of the groups from cohort 1:

> What's really different is that you guys [the group members] speak in plain English and you talk about what you mean...there isn't lots of

jargon. And that means you communicate more directly and you make more impact... The evidence from all of you seems to be that you've asked the right questions. And professionals are starting to say, whoa!

At least one of the group facilitators hoped that they could influence the wider research agenda:

We're quite pleased...we're hoping it will be picked up by a university, because it's a huge question. (Betty)

Several are also planning to write papers which they hope will be published in academic journals. Steve sums it up:

It's given me a fire and a passion that I want to move things forward; it's opened my eyes to a whole new world.

5. Inclusion, belonging and teamwork

One of the important outcomes has been the strong sense of inclusion that came from being part of a research team, or of the Pioneers group:

I've felt so comfortable and so welcome from the first off. Up here [my brain] it's working – that's down to you guys, bringing me into your group. (Steve)

I've only met one of you physically... But I feel as though I've known everyone for years. (Maq)

It was fantastic meeting the other DEEP groups... We're all very proud of it [our project] up here in Liverpool. (Paul)

We really got to know each other and got under the skin of each other, not in an annoying way, but just... And that was one of the best results that came out of it I think...was that interaction – smashing it was, yeah. (Chris)

The one thing I learnt...it's so much better to have help...that little piece of back-up is tremendous... Everyone here today, we're all working as a team together... We need to collaborate; there's plenty of intellect

People with Dementia at the Heart of Research

here, and plenty of innovation...to really get stuck in and really solve the problems. (Paul)

We'll end up being the best bloomin' network in the world. 'Cos we know what we're doing, there's lots of us. (Brian)

It was very interesting doing it...hearing different people's opinions and points of view...eye opening. (Sue)

It's something new for all of us, so I just feel proud of myself, that I've been part of the team; we've done this fantastic research all together.

I think we valued everybody's opinion, and everybody's got a different problem so you could put that across and everybody listened and understood. We have to share it, don't we? Everyone was able to share what they wanted to put in the questions.

I think it has felt like teamwork and everyone's brought really different opinions, and experiences and skills, and that's made it a richer project.

We all got involved, and we all got on well together, which is really good.

Everybody was very respectful – even when they had a difference of opinion, it was, 'How do we get that in?' People were listening to each other. There was a lot of respect there.

I think being honest as well, with the survey questions, and with each other – that's the great bit, isn't it? So that we can trust each other.

I felt like we were all equals: there was no one on a higher level than anyone else. Me personally, I felt that we were all one team, all equal, and that's how I have felt throughout this process.

Many of the DEEP researchers spoke about their sheer pleasure in doing this work, using words such as 'laughs' and 'fun', 'joy' and 'energy'. It seems that the process of coming together to share varied experiences and responsibility for a group task was at least as important as the research outputs themselves. Mhari was one of the original Pioneers.

Although she had to bow out later on due to ill-health, she reflected enthusiastically on the joy of being part of the programme:

> I'm chuffed to bits that I can be part of it all; it's really exciting... Just being here, having conversations about this – it's a winner for so many people... It would be great if everybody...could join the party. It's expanding all the time...hopefully things will broaden out for everybody. (Mhari)

In summary, Dementia Enquirers has built the confidence of DEEP groups to lead their own research projects. People with dementia in these groups surprised themselves with what they achieved in their research project. When they started out they were quite nervous. But they shared ideas and skills and asked for help when they needed it. Together they became dementia researchers.

CHAPTER 7

What Does This All Mean for the Academic Community?

Dementia Enquirers has brought back the passion that has been battered out of academia. (Dr David Crepaz-Keay)

Chapter summary

In this chapter, we show the vital and unique role that academics can play in:

- helping to 'shift the power' and democratize research
- thinking about research hierarchies differently
- inviting people with dementia to choose their own topics for research
- supporting people with dementia to be 'in the driving seat'
- making everything in research more accessible
- approaching ethics from the perspective of people with dementia
- encouraging people with dementia to co-author reports and articles with them
- being more open to different types of evidence.

We also describe the learning from the programme which is most relevant to research funders. We discuss how they can play an influential role in helping people with dementia to move into the driving seat by:

- working with people with dementia to assess funding applications

- opening up funding streams to people with dementia
- working with people with dementia to draw up a list of priority areas or questions for research
- promoting the DEEP-Ethics Gold Standards
- funding a sustainable 'infrastructure'.

Shifting the power[1]

We are not undermining the wonderful work researchers do: we're saying we can bring a different and unique approach to research. (Wendy)

Change is happening. Funders generally do have expectations of involvement and PPIE ('patient and public involvement and engagement') is a solid expectation for most. It's great when academics invite people with dementia onto their new project's research interest group or advisory group (please not just *one* person with dementia – or worse, just carers as proxies!).

But for budgetary and organizational reasons, universities sometimes go with the easy option. And in most PPIE and co-production projects, there is still the question 'On whose terms are we working?' It rarely feels like the partnership which the title implies. The quality of a lot of PPIE is still debateable, with many people with dementia being critical of the more tokenistic efforts of some research projects. As part of Dementia Enquirers, we have set out Gold Standards on PPIE and co-production (see Chapter 8). These can be delivered to a very high quality, and people with dementia are highly favourable about these approaches when they are done well. However, the involvement of people with dementia is not static. As people grow in confidence, their expectations about involvement increase. Involvement encourages more involvement. People with dementia leading research becomes a logical next step.

When we invited people with dementia to help us to shape the programme, they immediately rejected the traditional term 'research interest group' and chose instead their own name of 'Pioneers', as explained in Chapter 1. What is more, the academics who volunteered

---

1   This section draws heavily on an article by the Pioneers (Berry *et al.*, 2019).

their support for the programme became 'advisors' or 'allies'. Their advice was enormously valuable – but the power had definitely shifted. And to sustain and embed that, we needed to work very hard to ensure that all the processes used were co-designed to be accessible, while remaining robust and effective.

We hope that Dementia Enquirers will add some thinking and learning to the way that people with dementia are involved in research. We hope we have shown how hard we all need to think about the power within the group and the importance of accessibility. People with dementia are not downplaying the enormous expertise in the field of research, but at the moment, they feel they are always walking through the doors of researchers. Now they are asking researchers to walk through *theirs* and to turn research on its head by starting from *their* point of view.

In dementia research, co-production is not good enough. We have shown how people with dementia can *drive* the research (albeit with access to other support and expertise). It comes down to *power*. In a sense, the programme seeks to democratize research. We hope we have helped to shift the nature of knowledge and evidence, and the way we see the world. What we did before was not working for anyone.

> What I'd love to see is the whole academic world become much more open and accessible to people living with dementia, as members of that research community, so that we can all start to generate knowledge together. (David Crepaz-Keay, advisor)

Academics have a key role to play in increasing the skills and knowledge of people with dementia; putting ownership, control and power into their hands; and supporting them to lead their own research. They can help to challenge or reverse power imbalance, turning on its head the traditional approach of people with dementia often 'giving' their lived expertise to universities.

Starting from a different place

Lay people – including people with dementia – will never replace, or seek to undermine, the skills and experience of academics. However, academics do have much to learn from the Dementia Enquirers programme in terms of working differently with people with dementia. Dementia Enquirers has addressed the problem of positionality head-on, asking, 'Who has a stake?'

One of the Pioneers, George Rook, has said that, generally, academic researchers come up with the topics of research before asking people with dementia to participate:

> It's looking at something they've thought of, rather than something we've thought of... When we choose the subject to research, it's gonna be a subject we care about, and that matters to us.

Academic research can be seen by people with lived experience as 'very obscure' and 'at a distance from reality'. Agnes has also explained:

> I've been involved in professional research – [it focuses on] very obscure questions. And I've thought, what difference will this make to people with dementia?

> Academic researchers tend to have a formula about how they generate research questions. People with dementia aren't bound by that, so what they actually ask are the questions that matter to them. (David Crepaz-Keay, advisor)

Academics and funders can support people with dementia to identify and focus on topics for research which are of relevance to their own experiences – and about which they can feel passionate. The Dementia Enquirers programme has meant 'focusing on things that happen to us'. This has highlighted how the research questions that people with dementia generate can be different from the existing research agenda. They are based on lived experience – on topics that will make a real difference in people's lives, and which reflect day-to-day struggles and social barriers.

Academics and funders must take responsibility to find out what these topics and questions are – and to accord these at least as much priority as their own interests.

Supporting, not leading

The Dementia Enquirers programme has also shown that people with dementia can lead their own research projects – both drawing on previous life skills and learning new ones to explore the questions that most interest them. Controlling the research and leading the way not only gives people with dementia a huge boost in confidence, but also gives research an invaluable new lens.

But being in the driving seat of research doesn't mean that they have to do everything themselves. It is pretty obvious that people with dementia will have varying (and probably fluctuating) amounts of energy, skill, research experience, time and cognitive ability. Academics have a key role to play in offering the support that may be needed. They have been very much involved in the Dementia Enquirers programme, and in many of the individual Dementia Enquirers research projects – but only as advisors. For example, they have helped with methodological questions, data analysis and sometimes, where relevant, obtaining ethical clearance.

To use a common expression from the disability rights movement, experts have been 'on tap, but not on top'. Or, as Wendy Mitchell puts it:

> Researchers will come through our door, instead of us entering through theirs... Using your academic experience, and our expertise by experience, then that's the winning formula.

So we need to think differently about research governance and hierarchies. For example, whereas a formal advisory group can disempower people with dementia if it is not carefully managed, adopting the model of a small and very flexible consultation group of 'respectful friends' allows total control over how they make use of the expertise available.

> Not only do we have a wonderful music piece, but we have a fantastic report with some really solid findings. Also a really good insight into how it is for people living with dementia to lead their own research projects. And I think that's a really powerful piece of evidence that we now have...what it's like for people with dementia to lead on these kinds of projects. (Jack Fackley, student supporter to Ashford Phoenix group)

Accessibility

When academics make the language and processes of research more accessible, this demystification helps everyone – including academics!

> I think if they used more plain language, and not all the academic language, it would make it easier for us to understand as well. (Dory)

Our co-produced resources *How To Do a Research Project* and *The Dementia Enquirers Gold Standards for Ethical Research* (Innovations in Dementia, 2023a, 2023b) are two examples of how this can be done.

We have also demonstrated how people with dementia can successfully analyse and select proposals, based on criteria they have chosen together; how they can deliver or co-deliver engaging presentations about research findings; and how they can write or co-write research reports. To achieve all these things, we had to reinvent and simplify ways of working *with* people with dementia.

Ethics

The work on *The Dementia Enquirers Gold Standards for Ethical Research* (Innovations in Dementia, 2023b) has highlighted that ethics permeate everything – it's so much more than just getting a proposal through a committee.

The feedback we have received by people who have used the Gold Standards is excellent, and will hopefully encourage others to apply them in their own work. Academics at the University of Stirling have piloted the Standards with students on their MSc course and have given us valuable feedback. They say that the tool is clear, easy to understand and 'jargon free'. It has helped the students to 'translate' the academic papers they read into the real world – and to see how to put the principles of ethical research into practice. It also encouraged them to think about their projects in a much more participatory way: that is, to think about working with people with dementia in the planning and design of their projects much more than they might otherwise have done. The Standards have additionally helped students to think about how they might plan out their fieldwork activities, what they would need to do to make sure their projects were ethical, and how they might best interact with people with dementia as participants in their research. The guidance on issues of capacity and consent was found to be particularly valuable, as these are often difficult issues for students to grasp.

The mini-internships and masterclasses mentioned in Chapter 2 also generated excellent feedback, in particular with regard to the Gold Standards:

I have learned so much from your comments already. Thank you all very much for your time and sharing your personal insights.

I used the example written in the Gold Standards – really helpful. And I referred to the Standards in the form for the ethics committee.

I think dementia is leading the way in involvement. Research in diabetes wouldn't have people with diabetes at ethics committees. You are pioneers!

I think this is a brilliant way to ensure that the research carried out is indeed meaningful. From a researcher's point of view, it's not always the top priority, so having a group of Pioneers to push forward this agenda really makes the difference for the field.

This has been so useful. I really appreciate you all giving your time to speak to us. And it's given me lots to think about for how I go about doing my own questionnaires and focus groups, and making sure these are enjoyable for people living with dementia to be part of. I would love to do co-research after my PhD.

It's been incredibly valuable. I will particularly take confidence in challenging ethics panels when trying to push through more accessible documentation, as opposed to accepting the standard, lengthy, jargon-filled documents.

This session was really useful for students and staff – thank you very much Pioneers. Your guidance on ethical dementia research is a fantastic tool and will be incredibly helpful for anyone designing a research project and thinking about ethics approval. (Dr Richard Ward, Senior Lecturer in Dementia Studies, Faculty of Social Sciences, University of Stirling)

Thanks to all the Pioneers who came to speak to our students. It's definitely inspired them as they continue with their studies...and, more importantly, I think you'll have encouraged them all to think about their future professional work in much more inclusive and participatory ways. (Dr Grant Gibson, Lecturer in Dementia Studies, Faculty of Social Sciences, University of Stirling)

The Gold Standards will be incredibly helpful in how we improve the quality of our dementia steering group in Humber and North Yorkshire. I will also share this with all members. I would love for you to present this to one of our next steering groups too if you could. (Gemma Willingham-Storr, Humber Coast and Vale Health and Care Partnership)

Co-authorship

Co-authorship of papers is something that academics should also be proactive about – though it may require the development of new skills on their part. A great example from the programme is how the paper co-produced by the Pioneers and Professor Tom Shakespeare (Davies *et al.*, 2021) was co-authored. We believe this to be not only exemplary, but also entirely replicable.

The following excerpts from that paper describe the process used so successfully:

This is a co-authored paper, led by people with dementia at all times, in which all participants had an equal say, and where no one was in charge. It is not research conducted by an academic with, let alone on, people with dementia.

The working method was that meetings were held during the Coronavirus lockdown, on Zoom. Tom facilitated the discussions, recorded the conversation and also took notes. As people talked, he was able to insert their contributions into the developing text. Wherever possible he used their words and phrases, both as direct quotations, but also as the connecting text woven into the narrative of the paper. Then at the next meeting, he shared the draft with the group, so that others could see what they had said, and make changes. He also had separate Zoom discussions with two of the local DEEP [Dementia Engagement and

Empowerment Project] groups who were doing research projects. Tom was committed to listening to the group. For example, he had suggested putting the quotations from people with dementia in italics. But then it was pointed out to him that people with dementia found italics much harder to read. Agnes told him to 'put a wee note to explain why you didn't use the normal approach', using the italics example. The listening, sharing and checking ensured that it was truly co-production. The resulting paper is unusual in including long quotations from authors. This has been Tom facilitating people with dementia to speak for themselves, as researchers, not as research participants. Everything has been checked, modified and approved by all the authors.

The result, although apparently time-consuming, turned out to be very efficient. Short, intense days of interaction produced good results. The Dementia Pioneers found the work very exhausting, but were proud of what had been achieved: 'It would have taken others many months and many more meetings to achieve what we achieved today'. Some of the sense of urgency behind the work was a result of the feeling that many had that they were going to lose their cognitive capacities at some future point, so they wanted to get ahead now. Although the meetings were informal and fun, the Pioneers did not lose sight of the fact that they were trying to be more professional. They wanted to be able to break some academic rules, but they were willing to play by others, such as those governing this journal article. Ultimately, they were keen for people to read what they had to say, so that it might lead to changed perceptions of people with dementia by academics and clinicians. As Howard said: 'Too often we're getting a diagnosis and told we're incapable, but we're turning around and saying: "We are capable, and we can do the things that academics can do".'

The nature of evidence

The 26 projects funded by the Dementia Enquirers programme have also raised the thorny question of 'What is evidence?' One of our principles is that experiential knowledge needs to be taken as worthy of influencing research. This kind of knowledge is by no means lesser than the knowledge of other stakeholders. But it is the case that *all* knowledge, including the knowledge of academics, is *partial* – we are trying to find the whole picture. Dementia Enquirers has opened up new questions for research, and piloted new ways of answering those questions.

As explained in the article co-authored by the Pioneers (Davies *et al.*, 2021), the projects have tended to focus on practical action research rather than on traditional, more theoretical research. Several of the Dementia Enquirers were concerned that their questions were too practical to be genuine research. George Rook explains:

> I think academic researchers might regard what we do, certainly in this Pioneers project, as not really doing research. It's finding out some stuff, but research sounds as if it ought to be more difficult, more obscure and abstract. But we need to make the point that just finding out how much Admiral Nurses know about DEEP and how much DEEP know about Academic Nurses *is* research. There are many different types of research.

Wendy Mitchell agrees:

> We're being questioned about whether it's research, because some researchers are feeling threatened, as if we're questioning their expertise. But we're not. We're redefining the broadness of research. We're actually researching what we want to, what we think is important.

One of our advisors, David Crepaz-Keay, reassured us on this by introducing us to the concept of epistemic injustice (Fricker, 2007). This tells us that evidence is treated differently depending on who generates it, and that some knowledge makers are disadvantaged because of who they are. Liabo and colleagues (2022, p.2) explain further:

> Public involvement can increase the epistemological resources of researchers, and contribute to research that is fit for purpose and has high external validity...experiential knowledge...gained through living with health and illnesses, and receiving healthcare...arises when these experiences are converted, consciously or unconsciously, into a personal insight.

When this knowledge from the lived experience is accorded lower value, it creates epistemic injustice. You can watch a discussion we held in 2023 about epistemic injustice.[2]

As the Kent Forget-me-nots[3] reported:

> The students that have helped us have seen considerable growth in their abilities and knowledge during this enquiry, and the ability to foster said growth is one of the reasons enquiries such as these are so important.

ECREDibles – a partnership between a DEEP group and a university

One of the projects funded in the final year of Dementia Enquirers was ECREDibles. The group will eventually be open to all those living with dementia in Scotland, although it started with around ten members. They set out to find out if and how a DEEP group, hosted by people with dementia, could work effectively in symbiosis with a Scottish university group at the Edinburgh Centre for Research on the Experience of Dementia (ECRED).[4] The point of the project was to facilitate people living with dementia to lead their choice of research subject/projects from within an academic institution. Together they wanted to investigate and develop research ideas; empower more people living with dementia to benefit from university experiences, research and conference opportunities; and create more power and control within academic relationships. ECRED, as the academic project partner, brought the 'inside knowledge' of how to support ethics applications, and access research tools unavailable to those outside academic institutions.

The report describes the first few months of the ECREDibles partnership. The group met regularly, at least monthly, online and in person, in order to support each other and benefit from the university and project team's inspiration and knowledge, together with the knowledge and inspiration of the experts by experience. Working together, they decided on research questions and projects and pooled their resources to achieve their aims.

---

2   www.youtube.com/watch?v=C68Gr8PPhn0
3   https://dementiaenquirers.org.uk/wp-content/uploads/2021/10/10106a_de-report-forget-me-nots-october-2021.pdf
4   www.ed.ac.uk/health/research/centres/ecred

The group members each had specific skills. Methods were decided by the wider group as a project was planned, making full use of the benefits of working in partnership. The group enabled experts by experience to work in full and equal partnership with academic partners to achieve their aims:

> I like the idea of working in a symbiotic relationship – otherwise what's in it for us? It places us as experts, as the alumni. (Agnes)

> Why can't we choose our own research subjects? (Martin)

> Personally, I think this is a brilliant idea... I think the notion of having a body that could lend some credibility/degree of formality to our 'lived experience' is excellent. (Willy)

The other partners have been equally positive:

> We want to challenge traditional 'top down' hierarchies and promote new ways of working where those with dementia are making choices and being active in research. The ECREDibles is a ground-breaking project that is making this happen.

> The ECREDibles disrupts existing university structures and this is what we want...This creates challenges, but they are important challenges that mean we are working towards a more equitable future.

> It has given me the opportunity to engage more fully in the experience of dementia as someone who doesn't have a diagnosis of dementia, and learn significantly from those with lived experience. The ECREDibles has also provided an opportunity to share the skills I have developed as a researcher with them, which has been a great learning experience for me.

> It means that we always have the voice of lived experience at each meeting.

> I believe the ECREDibles are beginning to push the boundaries of less inclusive systems, or standard ways of doing things.

The group hope to learn more formal academic research skills and net-working with academic teams, being able to choose research subjects. People new to campaigning and research will benefit from the lived experience of existing campaigners and researchers.

Funding research differently

Almost all research funders now have expectations of involvement of people with dementia in these projects. But we would argue that this can still sometimes be tokenistic and regarded as an add-on, both in terms of budget and of actualization. Yet, as we have shown, this can be a huge opportunity missed, and it is so important to think more broadly and creatively. We set out below some of the learning from Dementia Enquirers which we hope will influence funders.

Working with people with dementia to assess funding applications

During the course of the programme, nearly 30 funding applications have been assessed by people with dementia (the Pioneers). We consider this to be a real achievement from which others can learn. Setting criteria, designing application processes and deciding which proposals to fund have all been achieved through genuine co-production. We made a short film where the Pioneers talk about the process of reviewing the first cohort of research proposals – including the importance of being in a relaxing and energizing venue.[5] These are some quotes from the film:

> We didn't always agree but we debated about it…and voted accordingly. But I think it was the honesty – we felt so comfortable with one another that we could speak from the start. (Agnes)

> I loved the way that we just followed our own hearts. (Tracey)

> It has worked for all of us… I really enjoyed it. (Mhari)

One of our advisors, Dr Rosie Ashworth, also found it 'really humbling

---

5   www.youtube.com/watch?v=KX2NiBhjhhY&t=5s

to have that role completely reversed – there was a real excitement about what could be achieved'.

Opening up funding streams to people with dementia

Although a few of the projects we funded received up to £10,000 (usually when more than one DEEP group was involved), most had no more than £5000. Some asked for less, and others returned unused funds. This shows how little is needed for people with dementia to set up their own modest research projects.

Having said that, the programme has also showed that a certain level of infrastructure and support is needed to help projects succeed. This might be in the form of administrative support, travel sponsorship, academic partners, unpaid time from group facilitators, and the light-touch mentorship from Innovations in Dementia. These costs-in-kind varied a lot but they do need to be taken into account.

We would love to see funders opening up funding streams to projects led by people with dementia, following the leadership of the National Lottery Community Fund with Dementia Enquirers.

Working with people with dementia to draw up a list of priority areas or questions for research

The programme allowed/enabled the DEEP groups to choose any topic as their research questions – we decide not to set any parameters at all. The resulting list highlighted that people with dementia choose different topics from academics. It also suggests to us that funders could benefit from working alongside people with dementia when they set up their own funding programmes.

Promoting The Dementia Enquirers Gold Standards for Ethical Research

Academics must show their respect for what people with dementia have produced or co-produced. They can (and we think should!) be guided by *The Dementia Enquirers Gold Standards for Ethical Research* (Innovations in Dementia, 2023b) right from the start of drafting their proposals; before submitting to a funder; before submitting to a REC; and throughout the whole process of fieldwork, analysis, reporting and dissemination. We would also like to see funders suggest (or even require) that projects that apply for funding follow the Standards and/or meet with a panel of Pioneers to discuss their proposals in the context of the Standards.

Funding a sustainable 'infrastructure'

In order to sustain the momentum created by the Dementia Enquirers programme there will need to be more and longer-term funding for the requisite infrastructure. One example (already discussed above) that is being tested at a more local level is that of the ECREDibles, a group which has partnered with a university (ECRED at University of Edinburgh). Their report[6] describes in detail the learning that has been generated by this innovative collaboration and the adjustments that have had to be made, for example, creating more accessible guidance on funding and new systems for payments, enabling library access and allowing videos as a format for grant applications.

The testimony of the academics involved in this partnership is unequivocally positive:

> This is the first time that I have collaborated directly with those living with dementia to co-design research funding applications. This has been completely invaluable to me. It has enabled me to...work towards a future where all those with dementia have the opportunity to be research leaders.

> Dementia Enquirers have really put a flag in the sand, saying, 'This is your starting point now, and now you need to be better, you need to keep building on this.' I think it's so exciting to see people come together and want to learn about this... It has certainly given me that kind of motivation. (Dr Rosie Ashworth)

This pilot highlights the many benefits that can come from a genuine co-produced research partnership. However, there are things to consider and to have in place to make this type of research dynamic work. The Swindon Forget Me Not Centre research group have worked together on research projects since 2017, and have a well-established dynamic and

---

6   https://dementiaenquirers.org.uk/wp-content/uploads/2022/09/ecredibles-september-2022.pdf

team relationship. In their report[7] they have highlighted the importance of these issues:

- Both time and money are needed to form trusting relationships and to properly reimburse people for their input, time and energy.
- A lot of flexibility is needed: for people with dementia this (probably) will not be their full-time job, and university researchers need to respect this.
- It is also key that everyone understands who does what in the project. This can be established at the start but also requires constant 'checking-in', so that nothing is assumed.
- A key message is that funders need to be aware of these factors and enable them. This is often not the case in grants, where money and time are kept strictly limited.

The work of Dementia Enquirers has already led to a number of new opportunities for people with dementia to lead their own research. One example is a project on public transport and mental health, which was funded by Motability (see following) and led by the Mental Health Foundation (MHF). The latter invited the Pioneers to lead their own small study from the perspective of people with dementia (2022–23).

Case study: Motability research project

The Motability project was a good avenue to test out some of the approaches that have been developed by Dementia Enquirers. Following an initial group discussion about the impact of travelling on public transport, supported by an artist evaluator, we thought about how to carry out this piece of research. We agreed we should keep it simple and straightforward to achieve. We should be careful not to be biased in the way we asked questions (e.g. we shouldn't assume everyone has a negative experience of travelling). We discussed the type of questions we could ask other people with dementia to find out about the impact on their mental health of travelling on public transport. We created a long list of questions to think about. We

---

7   https://dementiaenquirers.org.uk/wp-content/uploads/2022/10/forget-me-not-october-2022.pdf

also talked about the possible methods we might use in our research – discussing the pros and cons of questionnaires, interviews and a 'feelings measurement'.

After the initial two meetings, we designed an information sheet and consent form, and then we focused on ethics. We applied the Gold Standards for Ethical Research to make sure that our project was ethical in its approach.

Next, we looked at the answers to the questions pertaining to dementia in the public opinion survey, and we talked about how we could encourage more people with dementia to complete our survey. We became more realistic about what we could do in the given time – and chose a questionnaire as our research method. We finalized the survey and launched it on SurveyMonkey on behalf of the group.

We then looked at the results so far from our survey and thought about what these results might mean. We discussed how it seemed that there were many issues underlying the psychology of asking for help – maybe location, stigma and life experience, for example.

In the final meeting, we looked at the final results from our survey. We were surprised at some, less so at others. Some made us feel sad. We discussed the best ways of presenting the results so they were accessible to people with dementia (bar charts and pie charts are good, word clouds are bad!).

Conclusions

Once you start doing this type of research – you can't go back. You see the value of having user-led involvement, having that lived experience. (Dr Rosie Ashworth)

All these ways of doing things demonstrate, as Dr Wendy Mitchell puts it, that 'there is another way' for those in the academic community who choose to accept the challenge:

To be more open to not going down the same routes as they've always done. To look at other methods. To look at other ways of involvement. And to question what they do at the moment, to question their processes.

As George Rook says:

What we're doing is proving that they can do it differently. We've done it our way, following the rules we need to follow, adapting where we need to. You can too, and it won't diminish your research.

And the final word comes from Mhari McLintock, who was an active Pioneer for the first part of the programme until her health declined:

You can turn everything upside down...in a good way.

Building on the legacy of Dementia Enquirers: Ideas for academics

How can academics carry forward the learning from this programme? Drawing on learning from Dementia Enquirers, they can go beyond PPIE or even co-production and use our 'driving seat' model. They can invite and support people with dementia to:

- choose their own research priorities
- decide if, how and when they use the expertise of academics and advisors
- select methods which they feel comfortable with
- help make all processes and information as accessible as possible
- co-author papers with people with dementia
- help them express what is ethical and unethical from their perspective
- show people with dementia how valuable they find their experiential knowledge.

Building on the legacy of Dementia Enquirers: Ideas for funders

How can you, as a research funder, carry forward the learning from this programme?

- You are perfectly placed to set higher funding expectations about the involvement of people with dementia in research, promoting a driving seat model as well as PPIE and co-production. Research funders have a role in encouraging researchers to shift power and democratize research.
- You can encourage dementia researchers to use the Dementia Enquirers resources to plan and deliver their research, involving people with dementia from the very beginning.
- With most research funding being directed through academic institutions, there is a major barrier to people with dementia leading their own research. You could develop research funding streams that would enable people with dementia to take the lead in funding applications.
- Finally, you could ask applicants to show that they have applied the Dementia Enquirers Gold Standards for Ethical Research.

CHAPTER 8

Towards a New Model of Co-Research: 'The Driving Seat'

Research about us shouldn't be without us! (Dr Wendy Mitchell)

Chapter summary

Dementia Enquirers was set up to explore what it means for people with dementia to be 'in the driving seat' of research. We supported a number of groups of people with dementia to run their own research projects to find out if this was possible. Along the way, as it turned out, we have also challenged and tried to improve some of the broader aspects of the research process.

The learning from all this work has helped us to develop a new model of co-research with people with dementia, which we have called the 'driving seat' model. Additionally, our work has helped us to define and refine the essential components of high-quality co-production, where people with dementia and researchers 'share the driving seat'. There is a lot of overlap between the two models, but also some fundamental differences.

Introduction

In Chapter 1, we set out the background to why we developed the Dementia Enquirers programme. We discussed radical approaches to emancipatory research in the disability field, whereby people who use services (rather than professionals) are not just involved in research but have control over the research processes. We acknowledged that the involvement of people with dementia is often on the terms of academic researchers, and that research doesn't necessarily answer the kinds of questions that people with dementia are interested in. And we wondered if there was a next step – with the right support, could people with dementia lead their own research enquiries? Could they be in the driving seat of research?

In this chapter, we will present two models that can be used in good co-research with people with dementia. One is the co-production model (which we describe as 'sharing the driving seat' with academics [academics being a co-driver essential to making decisions]). The second is the driving seat model (people with dementia being solely 'in the driving seat' with advice [but not decision-making] from academics).

The co-production model – sharing the driving seat

High-quality co-production (and PPIE: 'patient and public involvement and engagement') in research has got many benefits, according to people with dementia. True collaborations between people with dementia and researchers can result in:

- a range of expertise in the same place, with a balance of lived experience and researcher skills and knowledge
- opportunities for learning and development of new skills for people with dementia
- access to larger funding streams and therefore opportunities for more research.

Our model sets out the six standards that make co-production a good experience for everyone, non-tokenistic and useful to the research. These are:

1. The lens of lived experience
2. Negotiated roles and involvement
3. A relationship of trust and respect
4. Dementia adjustments
5. Scaffolding
6. Shared values

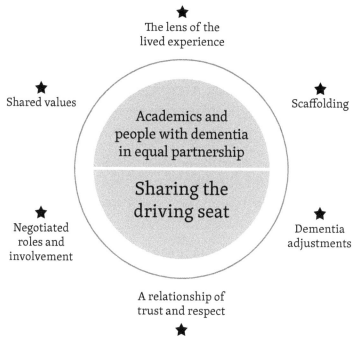

The lens of the
lived experience

Shared values

Scaffolding

**Academics and
people with dementia
in equal partnership**

**Sharing the
driving seat**

Negotiated
roles and
involvement

Dementia
adjustments

A relationship of
trust and respect

DEMENTIA ENQUIRERS GOLD STANDARDS FOR CO-PRODUCTION

From Dementia Enquirers, we know that the involvement of people with dementia is not static. As people grow in confidence, their expectations about involvement increase. Involvement encourages more involvement. Good PPIE encourages co-production. Good co-production might even lead to people with dementia being more in the driving seat of research, leading their own research studies.

The 'driving seat' model

Dementia Enquirers has been about increasing the skills and knowledge of people with dementia to lead their own research. Their lived experience puts them in a very good position to say what dementia research should be about and how it should be carried out.

People with dementia have also adapted research methods and frameworks to be more dementia accessible, and have developed new ways of working within traditional research systems such as ethics processes. It is about shifting the power and democratizing research.

It doesn't mean that people with dementia have to do everything – but that they maintain the lead throughout.

The driving seat model builds on the principles at the heart of PPIE and co-production – that is, that research is better when people who are recipients or subjects of research findings are involved. Consequently, our driving seat model has two additional standards to our co-production model:

1. People with dementia in control over the topic, the research question and the methods.
2. Liberation from rigid and inaccessible structures.

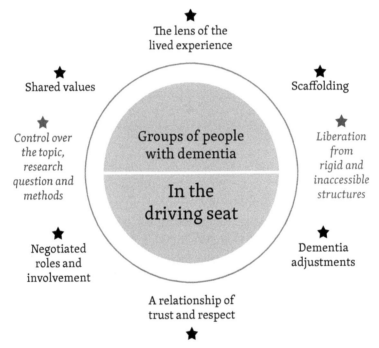

DEMENTIA ENQUIRERS GOLD STANDARD FOR THE DRIVING SEAT MODEL

The Dementia Enquirers Gold Standards for Co-research

We developed the Dementia Enquirers Gold Standards because we wanted to support (and encourage) researchers to think differently about the ways that they involve people with dementia in their research. We believe that academic researchers have their own roles to play in challenging or reversing power imbalances in research, turning on its head the traditional approach of people with dementia often 'giving' their lived experience to universities. These Gold Standards:

- are defined by people with dementia
- start from the assumption that co-research is the place you want to be and that you want to do it as well as you can
- use a disability rights approach, which is clear about the 'reasonable adjustments' that should be made
- are a starting point – in your co-research with people with dementia you will generate, together, more principles and practicalities that are specific to you and your research
- progress towards people with dementia being in the driving seat of research.

Standard 1: The lens of lived experience

How can we acknowledge the importance of adding the voices of people with dementia into research processes? As researchers (with and without dementia) we will:

- Publicly acknowledge the importance of a co-research approach in our research; include this in our research websites, publicity materials and funding reports; say it regularly to people with dementia.
- Look at every aspect of our research, including anticipated work; write a co-research plan for each part of the research in collaboration with people with dementia; keep adjusting this together as the research goes on.
- Not expect people with dementia to be representative of other people with dementia, even though they will often bring with them the experiences of other people; add numbers to our co-research activities to build a range of diverse experiences.
- Create a feeling of equality within our research team, with people with dementia being as important as researchers, and others; we all bring a partial view of the world, and benefit by joining these partial views together.

Standard 2: Negotiated roles and involvement

How will we negotiate and agree roles based on people's different interests, skills and knowledge? As researchers (with and without dementia) we will:

- Find out the skills and interests that people with dementia bring. There will probably be some surprises!
- Offer opportunities for people to learn about research processes. This can be through written information, a seminar or training. Think about the most appropriate ways of providing this learning – people differ in their learning styles and preferences.
- Share stories around our research team. This can help inspire people about roles and opportunities available that they haven't taken up yet. A regular accessible newsletter is a way of doing this.
- Share regular reminders about the research. As the 'jobs' stack up it can be easy to forget the focus and purpose of the research.
- Keep talking about the things that people might like to get involved in. These can change as people become more confident or their personal circumstances change.
- Acknowledge what has changed because of co-research; keep a record of the co-research activity and any action/change that has happened. If we keep adding to this list it becomes a visible, and potentially public, record of our whole approach.

Standard 3: A relationship of trust and respect

We need to take steps to make sure that positive feelings arise in co-production – for everyone! Feelings of 'trust and respect' can be difficult to measure, so think about how we will 'know' it's there. As researchers (with and without dementia) we will:

- Let go of some of our learned 'professional' behaviour! Relax, share stories, be open and warm, listen, smile and laugh.
- Do what we say we will do; let people know we have done it; provide feedback about what has changed.
- Aim to create the best environment for co-research; find out from people with dementia what this looks like (and take a look at Standards 4 and 5).

- Hold the co-research space, or make sure someone else does this. People with dementia need to feel safe and secure that they are noticed, can speak, are being listened to and any concerns are acknowledged. Use props to help with this such as the 'I Want to Speak' cards that have been designed and promoted via DEEP (the UK Network of Dementia Voices).[1]
- Notice people who are quieter. Are there ways that we can draw them in? Would direct questions help? Or could we speak with them outside a main meeting?

Standard 4: Dementia adjustments

What adjustments can we make that ensures co-research is a good experience for people with dementia? As researchers (with or without dementia) we will:

- Write information about the project in a dementia-accessible way. Where possible, try and write the same information in the same style for everyone, rather than 'special' information for people with dementia. (Innovations in Dementia (2023c) has produced advice about writing clearly for people with dementia.)
- When running meetings, send out reminders beforehand and on the day; keep processes as simple as possible.
- Draw on guidance from DEEP (Dementia Engagement and Empowerment Project) about running face-to-face meetings, online meetings and travel plans (Innovations in Dementia, 2022).
- Keep meetings to an hour where possible. If a meeting is longer, make sure that breaks are factored into the agenda.
- Limit agenda items at meetings to one or two main discussions.
- Take it slowly; don't speak too fast; leave lots of space for people to speak; notice people's body language, which may show they want to speak or are trying to organize their thoughts.
- Translate and modify standard research systems to be as accessible as possible; strive for clarity in every aspect, not least in language (no acronyms, jargon etc.)

---

[1] www.dementiavoices.org.uk/deep-resources/resources-for-deep-groups/resources-for-meeting-and-gatherings

- Write up accessible minutes of meetings straight away and send them out to people within a few days.
- Chat to people after events and meetings to find out what the experience was like and what might need to change in the future.
- Find out from people with dementia the personalized adjustments that will help them to participate in this role.
- Give time, time and more time. Things will take longer, but meetings may need to be shorter. Ensure that managers and funders are conscious of the extra time (and therefore maybe budget) needed for high-quality co-production with people with dementia.

Standard 5: Scaffolding

What kind of behind-the-scenes, sometimes invisible, support will make people with dementia feel safe and secure in their role? As researchers (with or without dementia) we will:

- Carry the load on behind-the-scenes administrative support, such as travel, venues, appointments, arranging meetings, drafting and keeping in touch, all negotiated and agreed at the start, and ongoing (this has been described as 'Looking after us, taking the strain off us').
- Mentor and provide tailored support for any individual who needs it.
- Keep negotiating and making adjustments to how every member of the team works; be prepared to be flexible.
- Have high but realistic expectations of each other – encouraging regular two-way communication.
- Visualize the 'scaffolding' that needs to be provided to keep co-production working well (checking the nuts and bolts and Platforms regularly, tightening them up).
- Help to make research methods accessible and manageable by using the guide *How To Do a Research Project* (Innovations in Dementia, 2023a).

Standard 6: Shared values

Thinking about shared values provides the foundations for co-prod-uction. Making these explicit can help in the sharing of power. As researchers (with or without dementia) we will:

- Talk together about what is important to people.
- Create together a list of the values that connect us. It might take a while of working together to identify these, and what this might mean for the work.
- Return to our values at regular intervals; be explicit about how these values interact with our co-production work.
- Pay people with dementia for their time. This acknowledges the value of the role they play in research co-production.

Standard 7: People with dementia in control over the topic, the research question and the methods

People have full control (or at least as much control as they want). This ensures that research is about the things that *they* identify as most important. Their lived experience puts them in a very good position to say what dementia research should be about and how it should be carried out. As researchers (with or without dementia) we will:

- Encourage people with dementia to think about what is impor-tant to them in their lives. What questions do they have? What would they like to know more about? What issues do they spend time discussing?
- Use group discussion to help to centre people on the topics that they think are 'most important'.
- Support people with dementia to turn their research interests into a research question – by introducing a question mark.
- Help people to map the kinds of roles they might like to have in the delivery of the research. What skills and interests do people have? Who would like to learn new skills?
- Provide the scaffolding to help people take on a research role. This might be mentoring, accessible training, removing jargon and creating accessible summaries. These can go a long way to helping people to feel confident in their researcher role.
- Enable people with dementia to 'see' the whole research plan

– and identify the range of ways people could take over the driving seat at different points and throughout the whole research journey.

- Keep returning to the concept of the driving seat – how in control of the research are people with dementia feeling? What needs to change so that people with dementia retain ownership and are leading the research?
- Remember that being in the driving seat of research doesn't mean that you have to do everything yourself. Teamwork and support (scaffolding) can really help.
- Be an enabler – allow people with dementia to lead the way, calling on skills and experience as they need it, rather than the other way around.

Standard 8: Liberation from rigid and inaccessible structures

In Dementia Enquirers, people with dementia have had the opportunity to carry out their research differently. It can be liberating to step outside 'academic walls'. This liberation can relate to methodologies, processes, language, systems – all the ways of working which academics can adopt by default, but which are not necessarily suited to innovative and collaborative work. As researchers (with or without dementia) we will:

- Use the other resources of Dementia Enquirers to support a shift in the ways that research is carried out. Lots of researchers are referencing these resources in their funding applications and ethics applications.
- Use the Dementia Enquirers Gold Standards on Ethical Research to ensure our research is ethical from the perspective of people with dementia (not just to jump through the hoops of ethics approval).
- Take every opportunity to converse and work with people with dementia. They will teach us and help us to move outside our 'academic walls'.
- Publish our co-research (with people with dementia of course) in peer-reviewed journals, and help to build a body of evidence.

Implementing the driving seat model

As you begin to work more equitably with people with dementia you will discover together new ways of working that suit everyone. The Gold Standards are written to be adapted and built on to make them the best fit for each research project. The most important thing is to keep talking with people with dementia. Share your research space and together you will continue to define and add to these Gold Standards in a way that is particular to your own research. At the heart of it are these principles:

- Make sure people with dementia are involved at every step of the way, especially as the research is being formulated.
- Provide the scaffolding. If this is an academic research team then you should do the adapting, not expect people with dementia to adapt to you.
- Be flexible in the way your research is carried out. Adapt systems, make writing and meetings dementia accessible, keep talking and find out what works best.
- Build trusting relationships with people with dementia based on agreed values.
- Be willing to do things differently.

Reflections on the two models of co-research

One of the strengths of the driving seat model is that it makes full use of all the skills that people with dementia can bring, and creates self-esteem and empowerment. People have full control (or at least as much control as they want). It also ensures that research is about the things that *they* identify as most important.

However, this model demands time, energy, skill and a lot of support. It relies on a conviction that this kind of involvement is essential to research. Until this is adequately supported, the model is unlikely to become widespread. However, this need for support should be seen as a goal, not a limitation.

The driving seat model can liberate us from rigid and inaccessible structures and systems. On the other hand, co-production brings the ease of working within existing structures and systems. It also means that academic know-how is on tap, as is access to research funding, ethics approval and publication systems – whereas, in the driving seat model, all these may be much harder to achieve, at least at present.

The driving seat analogy

It is worth reflecting at this point on the driving seat analogy. This has wound like a silk thread through the whole programme. Right from the start, it encouraged us all to think big and brave – and to challenge those aspects of doing research that were experienced as disempowering. As previously mentioned, we commissioned cartoonist Tony Husband to create an image for us which really captured these aspirations.

However, as the programme progressed, we found ourselves regularly questioning and trying to refine (or even replace) this analogy. First of all, it was obvious that only one person can sit in a driving seat – but this programme was about *groups* of people with dementia being in control. So maybe it was about *sharing* the driving seat rather than being the driver... But this will inevitably lead to an accident! Second, our learning from the 26 small projects was that not everyone in a group *wants* to take control in a leadership way. Some may *prefer* to take a back seat. But that doesn't mean that they are not contributing, or that they are not supporting the *group as a whole* to be in control. And third, there has always been acknowledgement that none of this could be done without the support of others – group facilitators and academics in particular.

So we have identified scaffolding as one of the key elements of both co-production and driving seat research – but this then becomes a metaphor about buildings, not cars! Maybe, it was suggested, it's about 'dual control'? Or maybe we are the 'sat-nav for academics'? But neither of these recognize that, in this model, it is people with dementia who have the overall control.

Perhaps in the end we have to simply recognize the limitations of the analogy, while celebrating its vivacity and courage. Until we come up with something even better, we'll be sticking with it!

CHAPTER 9

Reflections and Key Messages

I hope that researchers will look at the project, look at the book, look at the video, and say, 'We can involve people with dementia: they can be partners in research, not participants' – that we can go to them and say, 'What do you want researched? What is important to you?' (Howard)

The story of Dementia Enquirers is a proud story. It's still early days – and we know that real change and impact takes time to embed. What is happening with people with dementia at this point must be seen in the wider context of user involvement, emancipatory research and empowerment. It links back to the Charter of Needs and Demands drawn up over half a century ago by the mental health group Survivors Speak Out at their Edale conference in 1987 (Wallcraft & Sweeney, 2003). These movements share the broad progression from carers to service users, to real involvement, to co-production – and now to 'driving seat' leadership.

But although mental health survivors and people with disabilities have been 'walking this map' for over half a century, people with dementia must 'walk their own map'. Some things about dementia are different – not least the small window of opportunity that individuals often have, and the need for succession planning. But our programme has been scaffolded by a strong grassroots movement of people with dementia who want to be in control of their own lives and have agency in the world around them. Dementia Enquirers is an optimistic project, about what people with dementia can do, not what they can't, and it has started to build an alternative lens on living with dementia. It is about people with dementia reclaiming their experiences from academic researchers, asking different questions and sometimes getting different answers.

We believe that the learning from Dementia Enquirers can and should play a key role in shaping the process of future research – and in creating a new normality. Our work has destroyed perceptions about dementia, and shown what people are capable of when given encouragement and the right support. We've started lots of conversations. We've seen both researchers and people with dementia grow in confidence as they try out new approaches. We've provided a whole box of new tools so that people don't have to reinvent the wheel every time. We have laid the foundations for a new model of research which fully embraces the rights of people with dementia. 'Driving seat' research is vital if we are to understand what living well means.

People with dementia are teaching us how we can make the world a better place for them. This is history-shaping knowledge. What was happening before was not working for anyone – Dementia Enquirers has helped to shift the nature of knowledge and evidence, and the way we see the world. We have addressed the problem of positionality head-on, asking 'Who has a stake?' We have queried what evidence is. We have brought back the passion that many academics say has been battered out of academia. We've shown how research can be fun. We have found a new space in which research has been democratized. We have shown that there are many ways to be in the driving seat. We have demonstrated how people with dementia can play a leading role in research. We have shown the diversity of the experience of living with dementia – crossing social class, age and diversity (irrespective of the dementia diagnosis). Our projects have introduced new knowledge which has the potential to influence future research, policy, practice and attitudes.

If you make research easier it is better for everyone. The primary beneficiaries in this case are people with dementia, but there are many others too. Research becomes more interesting when it is more accessible. Our challenges throughout the programme to language, processes and ethics have pushed researchers to be more flexible and creative. Many of those who have been in involved in the programme have testified that the approach has really made them think – one has even called it 'career changing'.

And most important of all perhaps – people with dementia tell us that they feel they've been heard, listened to; that they feel their opinions matter, they still have worth, they are valuable.

Our ten key messages

1. People with dementia can lead their own research projects – drawing on previous life skills and learning new ones to explore the questions that most interest them.
2. This does not just apply to those who are the most 'able' or the least affected by dementia. The involvement is based on shared values and has been hugely diverse. Everyone has something to bring to the table.
3. The driving seat model goes beyond typical co-production because people with dementia are there right at the start – choosing the topic, the research question and the methods. And they are freer to do things differently, to venture beyond the usual paradigms.
4. Because they know what matters most to them, people with dementia share a determination and passion to make change happen and to overcome difficulties.
5. 'Driving seat' research is vital if we are to understand what living well means. The research questions that people with dementia generate are often different. They are based on lived experience – on topics that will make a real impact on people's lives.
6. Being in the 'driving seat of research' doesn't mean that you have to do everything yourself. Team work and support ('scaffolding') can really help.
7. Controlling the research and leading the way gives people with dementia (and their groups) a huge boost in confidence, and brings meaning to their lives.
8. Making the language and processes of research more accessible helps them, and everyone! This approach democratizes research.
9. People with dementia understand ethics and can come to considered judgements about capacity, consent and the risk of harm. They also bring a different perspective – which can make research more ethical.
10. Mainstream research processes, systems and governance need to be willing to adapt if people with dementia are to be included as equal partners.

What next?

Throughout the Dementia Enquirers programme, we have always been clear that the process – of finding out what it means to be 'in the driving seat' – is just as important as the findings of the projects themselves. We hope that what we have done, and the way we have worked, will open the eyes of the public, people with dementia and their supporters, as well as academics, research funders, research ethics committees, practitioners, commissioners and policymakers. We also hope that it may have helped to make closer connections with the wider disability world – we have learned a lot from co-production of research in the disability movement, and we hope that the disability movement will also find things to learn from us.

We hope that, in future, more facilitators will find the confidence to help their groups identify their own research priorities, apply for funding and carry out their own enquiries. Our work with universities and early career researchers has demonstrated how people with dementia can influence dementia education. We hope that groups will make closer connections with local academics and apply for funding as research partners.

We have also co-produced a whole range of resources within the programme which have the potential to improve the experience of people with dementia, whether as researchers, co-researchers, research advisors or research subjects/participants. And this can be at a global level. As Emily Ong (Dementia Alliance International) tweeted in 2022:

> We will need more of us with dementia in the driving seat of research and policy in different parts of the world, including in LMICs [lower and middle income countries].

> It does give us a voice, but it amplifies that voice. Those voices of people living with dementia through their research can impact all over the world, all over the globe. (Irene, Pioneer)

However, as this phase at least of the programme comes to an end, our call is for many more to pick up the baton and build on what we have achieved.

> The future looks brighter, and change will come. (George)

CHAPTER 10

Our Manifesto

The 'driving seat' model is still in its infancy, emerging from the work of Dementia Enquirers. We are relying on supportive allies to test it out and to help further develop the model. There is so much that every group can do! Here is our Manifesto.

DEEP groups and other involvement groups (people with dementia and group facilitators)

- Be confident to call for – and do! – research about the things that are important to you. What are your day-to-day struggles and social barriers. What are your hopes? The issues that you spend time talking about in your DEEP (Dementia Engagement and Empowerment Project) group are perfect for researching further.
- Be confident to tell people what helps you to get involved in research – and what hinders you.
- Find out what skills and life experience your members have that can help your group to do your own research.
- Try to make links with local universities and other allies who are interested in co-production.
- Be clear about the support you want/need – and the support you don't want/need.
- Encourage researchers to involve people with dementia better by telling them about Dementia Enquirers and the resources that have been co-produced.
- Make use of *How To Do a Research Project* (Innovations in Dementia, 2023a) to increase your confidence in a range of research methods.

- Promote *The Dementia Enquirers Gold Standards for Ethical Research* (Innovations in Dementia, 2023b) to all researchers with whom you have contact.
- Understand that doing research together on a topic for which you have a shared passion can be really bonding and enjoyable for a group.
- Get going with your own project!

Academics

Share power more comfortably. We have nothing to lose. You have so much to gain!

- Forge closer relationships with groups and networks of people with dementia.
- Encourage them to partner with you in a more equitable way, and as true co-investigators. In this way, you will help to challenge or reverse power imbalance, turning on its head the traditional approach of people with dementia 'giving' their lived expertise to universities.
- Support people with dementia to:
  - identify and focus on topics for research which are of relevance to their own experiences, and about which they can feel passionate.
  - decide if, how and when they use your expertise
  - select methods which they feel comfortable with
  - express what is ethical and unethical from their perspective
  - help make all processes and information as accessible as possible
  - co-author papers with you
  - deliver or co-deliver presentations about research findings.
- Adopt the model of a small and very flexible consultation group of 'respectful friends' (instead of a formal advisory group).
- Ensure that your language and processes are as accessible as possible: reinvent and simplify ways of working *alongside* people with dementia.

- Support people with dementia to analyse and select proposals, based on criteria they have chosen together.
- Show them how valuable you find their experiential knowledge.
- Be guided by *The Dementia Enquirers Gold Standards for Ethical Research* (Innovations in Dementia, 2023b) as you start to draft your proposals; before submitting to a funder; before submitting to a research ethics committee; and throughout the whole process of fieldwork, analysis, reporting and dissemination.
- Have courage to go beyond PPIE ('patient and public involvement and engagement') or even co-production and use our driving seat model.
- Practise the principle of scaffolding. For anybody with dementia who is involved in any way in your research:
  - Take time to find out each person's preferred ways of communication.
  - Give enough information (but not too much) to enable people to make an informed decision about whether to take part.
  - Keep everything as simple as possible – tailor your information so it is fit for purpose, for the audience and for the level of risk.
  - Use photos and other images if this helps to convey information.
  - Avoid overloading people with other (less accessible) information where it's not absolutely necessary.
  - Give people enough time to ask questions and make decisions.
  - Offer extra help to give informed consent. Elements such as visual props, Talking Mats and easy-read information can help people to understand and decide whether to be involved.
  - If people cannot sign a form, allow them to record their agreement on video or audio, or you could write a 'field note'.
  - Accept that consent is an ongoing and flexible process. Provide routine reminders and recaps (verbal, written or pictorial) that prompt people to reconsider and reflect on their involvement.
  - Remind participants the day before that they will be meeting with you, using the communication method that they indicate is best for them.

- Offer to help with travel plans, remote access, meeting people at stations and so on, if they need/want this to keep them safe.
- Make the schedule flexible to people's preferred time of day, and avoid days where other support might be limited (e.g. Friday evenings).
- Ensure that the research is conducted in a quiet, safe, private space and in keeping with the participant's wishes (if possible).
- For group discussions, think carefully about the venue – it needs to be peaceful, welcoming, fully accessible, well-signed, and with easy parking and transport links.
- Present all information clearly and accessibly, making reasonable adjustments as needed (including translation/ interpretation). Read out the guide on how to write accessible information for people with dementia (Innovations in Dementia 2023c).
- Speak at a steady pace and in simple (non-academic) language. Adapt to the person's own pace and preferred communication type and style.
- Explain research terms each time they are used (or use simpler alternatives) and avoid using abbreviations and acronyms.
- Avoid inappropriate exclusion of people, for example because of a diagnosis, deafness or language barrier. Take reasonable steps to be inclusive, for example offer translators, remote video conferencing or telephone where transport is not available or easily accessible. Avoid limiting your study to an upper age limit without good reason.
- Avoid over-taxing people's memory or communication skills. Always recap on previous conversations or interviews each time.
- Include enough breaks (e.g. for refreshments, quiet time, toilet and refocusing) because research involves a lot of concentration.
- Ask participants (and if agreed, their families or a trusted person whom they nominate) how they want feedback: at what points and in what ways? This may need to be rechecked.
- Provide a summary of the final report in simple, understandable language. Offer individuals a choice of what type of report

they want (e.g. a summary, two sides of key points or the full report). Reconfirm this at the end of their involvement.
- Ensure that payments and expenses are prompt and require minimal or no form-filling.

Research funders

- Design and resource specific funding streams for 'driving seat' projects, and reach out proactively to those who might want to apply.
- Set out your expectations of how people with dementia should be involved in research proposals, and their subsequent role in any funded research project.
- Encourage applicants to move beyond PPIE – and even co-production – and towards a driving seat model.
- Invite applicants to show that they have applied the Gold Standards (Innovations in Dementia, 2023b).
- Encourage researchers to draw on the resources available through the Dementia Enquirers programme, to plan and deliver their research, involving people with dementia from the very beginning.

Research ethics committees

- Accept that people with dementia can be in the driving seat of research.
- Make your own processes and language simpler and more accessible (though still in line of course with regulatory requirements).
- Encourage researchers to be guided by *The Dementia Enquirers Gold Standards for Ethical Research* (Innovations in Dementia, 2023b). This applies right from the start of drafting their proposals; before submitting to a funder; before submitting to a REC; and throughout the whole process of fieldwork, analysis, reporting and dissemination.
- Expect that research involving, or carried out by, people with

dementia must also use simpler and more accessible methods – and that these are not unethical.

- Accept that, if a project follows the Gold Standards, this is evidence that it is ethical (but this will not always mean that REC approval is not needed).
- Consider ways of involving people with dementia in REC decisions (you will need to adjust your processes).

Academic journals

- Consider your publishing criteria in relation to 'driving seat' projects and perhaps run special editions to promote them.
- Make your guidelines and processes fully accessible.

We believed we could...and we did. (Dory)

Summaries of Dementia Enquirers Projects

Ashford Phoenix (Kent): Therapeutic values of involvement in practical music-making

Ashford Phoenix are a group of like-minded people living with a diagnosis of dementia. They endeavour to improve understanding around dementia, both in the public arena and in NHS services. They meet monthly to discuss campaigning and dementia advocacy.

The group wanted to find out if people with dementia would benefit most from creating a piece of music by all learning a new instrument, rather than just being participants in music sessions. One member of the group had taken part in an online poetry course during the Covid-19 pandemic, and had noticed the significant impact creating poetry had on him. He wondered how music might affect him too. It is well documented that music has an impact on people living with dementia. However, this is often as passive recipients. The group wanted to turn this idea on its head and be in the driving seat of music-making.

The group planned, organized and took part in 12 music sessions, facilitated by a local musician. They learned the ukulele and composed a piece of original music. At each session, they completed before and after questionnaires relating to their mood and cognition. They also took part in focus groups at the beginning, middle and end of the project. One-to-one interviews were completed as well at the halfway stage of the sessions.

The results showed a positive effect immediately after sessions on group members' mood, but no change in cognition between sessions.

Focus group and interview data indicated that the project gave group members a focus, and de-stigmatized the idea that people with dementia cannot achieve goals or learn new skills.

The group felt that this project added to the literature on the impact of music on dementia, particularly due to the way in which they were at the forefront on the planning and reporting of the research. To read the full report visit https://dementiaenquirers.org.uk/wp-content/uploads/2022/11/ashford-phoenix-oct-2022.pdf.

Beth Johnson Foundation (Stoke-on-Trent) Project 1: Discrimination and dementia)

The Beth Johnson Foundation (BJF) in Stoke-on-Trent was one of the pioneers of advocacy, starting in 1989. In 1998, the dementia advocacy project was established, including this peer support and advocacy group. They aim to influence professionals from a grassroots perspective, by raising awareness about living positively with dementia.

BJF explored the question 'Does class, ethnicity or intellect affect the dementia pathway?' Members of the group had found that their different life experiences had a bearing on their own dementia pathway. The group used their own experiences to generate a long list of questions, which they narrowed down to five, reaching a consensus via discussion. Further focus groups took place, and the themes that emerged were discussed as a whole group – which led to findings and recommendations.

The group found that class, intellect and ethnicity all have a bearing on the dementia pathway. The impact of this can be both positive and negative. Class was perceived as employment and financial status, which can give people money to pursue hobbies and make necessary lifestyle changes. Class can also make you feel more confident to access support. Intellect was considered to be your education level and ability to access or understand information. Again, this can lead to more confidence to seek guidance and to speak out, including challenging ideas. Ethnicity can result in linguistic and cultural barriers. Dementia information is often published only in English, making it easily misunderstood or inaccessible to many.

The BJF advocacy group acknowledged that the dementia pathway is different for everyone. However, there are additional impacts of class, intellect and ethnicity in terms of how people adjust to their diagnosis and how others support them. An individualized response is needed and assumptions should be avoided.

To read the full report visit https://dementiaenquirers.org.uk/ wp-content/uploads/2021/05/beth_johnson_foundation_in_stoke-on-trent_report.pdf.

Beth Johnson Foundation (Stoke-on-Trent) Project 2: The pros and cons of living with dementia during Coronavirus

This Beth Johnson Foundation project was one of five projects funded in response to the Covid-19 pandemic. This funding stream acknowledged the restrictions that would impact the way that projects could be delivered. They interviewed each other to collate 'stories of Covid', resulting in a range of films.

To view the films visit https://dementiaenquirers.org.uk/projects/ beth-johnson-foundation-stoke-on-trent.

Beth Johnson Foundation (Stoke-on-Trent) Project 3: Exploring the experiences of dementia testing

For this project, the Beth Johnson Foundation (BJF) in Stoke-on-Trent group were interested to explore people's experiences of being tested for dementia. They were aware that they had all had different experiences, and there didn't seem to be any consistency.

The group decided to focus their research on the Addenbrooke's test as they are most familiar with this process. The Addenbrooke's Cognitive Examination is a screening test which considers attention, orientation, memory, language and visual and visuospatial skills. It is often used in the detection of Alzheimer's disease and fronto-temporal dementia. The group developed a questionnaire asking about the dementia testing process. Completed questionnaires were received from 42 people, and they conducted follow-up interviews with 23 people.

Most people said that no social history was taken during diagnosis. Over half had someone to accompany them during the test. Seventeen people did not have the test explained to them. People reported a range of different environments for testing, including a GP surgery, the hospital, a memory clinic in the community, and home. A lot of people felt negative after the test, including feeling dismissed, frustrated, unsure about next steps and patronized.

The group also spoke to staff at a memory clinic and a GP surgery to gather their views on the testing process. The group recommend that, whenever possible, people are tested at home, that the process is explained in advance, and a follow-up is offered to everyone.

To read the full report visit https://dementiaenquirers.org.uk/wp-content/uploads/2022/11/bjf-october-2022.pdf.

Budding Friends (Exeter): How Covid and lockdown has made me feel

Budding Friends is a group of people with dementia, carers and volunteers who meet once a week all year round. It is based around an allotment, with indoor activities taking place over winter. The Budding Friends project was one of five projects funded in response to the Covid-19 pandemic. This funding stream acknowledged the restrictions that would impact the way that projects could be delivered.

The group explored how the Covid-19 pandemic and lockdowns had affected the physical and mental wellbeing of people with dementia. They were very aware of the changes that members of their group had experienced, including moves into residential care. They interviewed people with dementia from the group, people with dementia from the local community, carers whose partners were in residential care and carers whose partners had died, some during the pandemic.

People with dementia described boredom, anxiety, isolation and deterioration of cognitive and physical abilities. Carers expressed a lot of distress, especially if their partner was in a care home. Visiting was minimal, and there were limited opportunities for true engagement. Carers felt that, if their partner had still been living at home, the decline would not have been so great.

The group concluded with recommendations relating to future pandemics for people with dementia, particularly in relation to the way the care home sector responds. To read the full report visit https://dementiaenquirers.org.uk/wp-content/uploads/2022/11/budding-friends-october-2022-1.pdf.

Deepness (Isle of Lewis): The necessary components of a dementia responsive training video

Deepness is a not-for-profit organization, run by and for people living with dementia and cognitive impairment. An offshoot is Deepness Dementia Media, a platform for tools around living well with dementia.

Deepness wanted to find out what type of video content works best for people with dementia. They were mainly interested in finding content to help people with dementia use technology. The group knew that much instructional video (e.g. on YouTube) is chaotic and wild and not dementia responsive.

Fourteen people with dementia took part in the project. They also acted as an expert advice group. The expert advice group were asked to watch three videos (made by Deepness) and then say which video was best for them, in response to a set of questions. The videos were of a young woman, an older woman and a middle-aged man. Discussions took place in a focus group.

The results showed that the content had to be clear, told slowly and said more than once. It was not important who the person in the video was. The group were a little disappointed that the focus group discussions resulted in a lot of agreement – i.e. a narrow range of views. They reflected that one-to-one interviews may have provided a much wider range of responses.

To read the full report visit https://dementiaenquirers.org.uk/wp-content/uploads/2021/05/deepness-on-the-isle-of-lewis_report.pdf.

ECREDibles (Scotland): Setting up a research peer support group

The ECREDibles is a new co-production group for people living in Scotland interested in research. It is led by people with dementia, working in partnership with the Edinburgh Centre for Research on the Experience of Dementia (ECRED). The group offer peer support to share ideas, information and inspiration about research projects and to co-produce their own research based on ideas from people with dementia.

The ECREDibles wanted to find out how a group of people with dementia could work in partnership with a university in order to lead research. This was an exploratory project, looking at whether a replicable model could be created to share across universities. The partnership with ECRED provides formal, contracted support to write research and funding bids, intern support hours and skills, staff support time, budget hosting and the advantage of a formal partnership with a university.

The group produced many recommendations about how people with dementia can be fully involved in this university partnership. Suggestions included rehearsal sessions on Zoom, recording minutes of meetings as audio files, shared files, sending reminders and providing travel support. This work is ongoing.

To read the full report visit https://dementiaenquirers.org.uk/wp-content/uploads/2022/09/ecredibles-september-2022.pdf.

EDUCATE (Stockport): The EDUCATE Echo Project

'EDUCATE' stands for Early Dementia Users Co-operative Aiming To Educate. It gives people with dementia a voice through involvement in training or speaking to others about their experiences of having dementia.

EDUCATE looked at how people with dementia used Amazon Echo Dot (Alexa) and what benefits or difficulties they experienced. EDUCATE describe the marginalization that many people with dementia experience following diagnosis. Alexa offers ways to keep people with dementia connected as well as keeping life regular, structured and independent. The group felt that technology such as Alexa has the potential to be useful for people with dementia.

Eighteen interested people with dementia were provided with an Alexa. People were supported to identify meaningful interests/tasks relating to the things they wanted. Individual support was given to people with dementia to explore Alexa and qualitative feedback was recorded about how people felt using it.

The project found that those who got the most benefit from using Alexa were those with poor short-term memory, but no language or visual problems. Those people with problems using or understanding language or meaning benefitted the least. Alexa could help with everyday tasks like cooking, answering the door, controlling the central heating, remembering appointments and taking medication. It was also helpful with activities and leisure pursuits. But support was often needed for account set-up, installation, troubleshooting and suggesting new functions.

The group concluded that Alexa has a lot to offer many people with dementia, but it is only as good as the support around it. Alexa needs to become more accessible and the necessary support systems need to be better understood.

To read the full report visit https://dementiaenquirers.org.uk/wp-content/uploads/2021/05/educate-in-stockport_report.pdf.

Forget-me-nots (Canterbury): The impact of Covid in relation to technology, relationships, coping and physical and mental health

Forget-me-nots is a group of older people with dementia. The aim of the group is to help people with dementia and to communicate to healthcare staff to help reduce the stigma surrounding it. Their project was one of five projects funded in response to the Covid-19 pandemic. This funding stream acknowledged the restrictions that would impact the way that projects could be delivered.

The group wanted to explore the impact of Covid-19 for members of their group. During the pandemic, the group had been forced to meet online, which had been a struggle for many members. They wanted to find out how best to support people with dementia during Covid-19, but also in the future.

The group created a list of questions for structured interviews looking at different aspects of people's struggles with the pandemic, including technology, relationships, coping strategies, challenges, physical/mental health issues, and any positives. People with dementia took on the role of interviewer. There was also a questionnaire of closed questions and tick boxes asking about use of technology before and after Covid-19.

The results showed that use of technology had increased since the pandemic and, although a lot of people required support, it was considered to be a real positive. Contact with professionals had reduced, although personal relationships were able to be maintained and even strengthened. People reported a decline in their dementia symptoms, although a range of coping strategies were shared.

The group concluded with recommendations relating to care and research. To read the full report visit https://dementiaenquirers.org.uk/wp-content/uploads/2021/10/10106a_de-report-forget-me-nots-october-2021.pdf.

Forget Me Not Centre research group (Swindon): Post-diagnosis dementia support

The Forget Me Not Centre research group was founded by three researchers living with dementia. Their goal is to improve the lives of people with dementia by valuing their expertise and lived experience. They want to influence everyone.

The group wanted to find out how people who had been diagnosed with dementia in the past four years experience their post-diagnosis care. They also wanted to explore ideas about how to improve post-diagnosis support. From previous work, they were struck by the different approaches to post-diagnosis support in different parts of the country (and even within the same city!). The group had all had a difficult time post-diagnosis and wanted to explore if things had changed.

Five focus groups were organized, with 18 people with dementia. Beforehand, people were sent a simple booklet explaining the topics that would be covered in the focus group. There was space so people could make notes under each topic. Because online meetings could feel impersonal, a packet of biscuits was sent to each participant to enjoy in the tea break.

Results included difficulty navigating (and finding out about) the benefits system, the postcode lottery of post-diagnosis support, a lack of support services (being left to 'get on with it'), the value of peer support, the perception that dementia is not treated equally, and feeling stigmatized.

The group made recommendations for improving dementia support. To read the full report visit https://dementiaenquirers.org.uk/wp-content/uploads/2022/10/forget-me-not-october-2022.pdf.

Great Camden Minds: Access to printed information as a person with dementia

Great Camden Minds is a dementia involvement and peer support group. They describe themselves as a 'friendly bunch' with an interest in making things in Camden more dementia friendly.

The aim of this project was to discover how easy it is to find information on dementia services in Camden for older people with dementia. The entire group found paper-based information on dementia important. The group were all over the age of 75, didn't use computers, smartphones or the internet, and often struggled with telephone calls. They noticed that it was becoming harder to get information, by themselves, about dementia. They lived independently and like to find things for themselves.

The group carried out a tour of local services over a three-month period. This included 15 GP surgeries, dentists, gyms, community centres and local libraries. They struggled to find any printed leaflets on local dementia services, help and support, or even references to dementia. The group found that there was a significant lack of printed information – leaflets, posters, flyers – on dementia in Camden.

They recommended that services develop more written information for people with dementia, and that this is accessible and relevant. They are working on an easy-read version of a leaflet that summarizes dementia services, help and support in Camden.

To read the full report visit https://dementiaenquirers.org.uk/wp-content/uploads/2022/11/great-camden-minds-nov-2022_v1.pdf.

Lifting the Cloud (Derby): Researching visitor attractions in Derby through the eyes of a person with dementia

Lifting the Clouds is a peer support group of people with dementia and carers. It keeps people engaged and reduces social isolation. They are passionate about raising awareness of dementia and trying to improve experiences for people with a diagnosis.

The group wanted to create a booklet that could help anyone with dementia who was visiting Derby as a tourist. This would be a guide to attractions and cover any difficulties they may experience which could impact their visit.

The group created a questionnaire which highlighted significant areas that could possibly be challenging for a person with dementia. Some people filled in the questionnaire during their visit; others took it home and filled it in later. At the end of a visit, the group also had a discussion about their experiences.

All of these results informed the development of a new booklet: *Derby Visitors Attractions: Through the Eyes of a Person Living with Dementia*. You can read the booklet at www.dementiavoices.org.uk/wp-content/uploads/2018/05/Derby-Visitors-Book-Pages-Web.pdf.

To read the full report visit https://dementiaenquirers.org.uk/ wp-content/uploads/2022/10/lifting-the-cloud-oct-2022-report.pdf.

Minds and Voices (York): Living with dementia with and without a care partner

Minds and Voices (York) is a fun, friendly and welcoming peer support group for people with dementia in the York area. They are keen to change people's perceptions of people with dementia. They say 'We still have a great deal to contribute and strongly believe that you CAN live as well as possible with dementia.'

Minds and Voices looked at the pros, cons and particular needs of those living alone with dementia and those living with a care partner. This was a conversation that unfolded often within group meetings, with different people having different preferences.

Minds and Voices carried out a literature review, a series of individual interviews and a focus group involving nine people with dementia in total – four people who lived alone and five who lived with care partners. They asked people to comment about their individual circumstances, and then to reflect on how they might feel if their circumstances changed.

They found that people who lived on their own felt they had many advantages, although loneliness was highlighted as a disadvantage. People who lived with a care partner enjoyed the company, fun and reassurance. However, they commonly encountered the frustration that dementia can bring to a relationship difficult.

Minds and Voices recommended that service providers and others should know more about people's individual circumstances. They should help people think ahead to if and when these circumstances change. They should not assume that someone living alone is in a risky situation. They advise that people with dementia talk (to each other) and also about the future.

To read the full report visit https://dementiaenquirers.org.uk/ wp-content/uploads/2021/05/minds-and-voices-in-york_report.pdf.

Our Voice Matters (Hartlepool): How community-based activities can have an impact on people living with dementia

Our Voice Matters is a peer support group of people living with dementia. They identify ways that Hartlepool can be more dementia friendly. They also spread the word about living well with dementia.

Our Voice Matters wanted to know what the impact of community-based groups was on people with dementia. People with dementia knew that they had thrived by being involved in different activities and groups in Hartlepool. They thought a lot of this success was down to encouragement at diagnosis, which gave them the confidence to start or join groups.

They created a survey and had group discussions with people with dementia to find out about the impact of being engaged in activities. They also created a survey for professionals to find out about their experiences of organizing activities in the community. The group found that attending group activities provided a range of benefits including: (a) making friends, (b) socializing, (c) having fun, (d) relaxing, (e) enjoyment, and (f) finding out about other things available in their area.

The results from people with dementia and professionals helped the group to create some top tips for people starting a group and those who are attending a group for the first time. To read the full report visit https://dementiaenquirers.org.uk/wp-content/uploads/2021/05/our-voice-matters-in-hartlepool_report.pdf.

Riversiders (Shrewsbury): Annual dementia reviews

Riversiders (Shrewsbury) is a peer support group run by people with dementia. In addition to being a group where members support each other and chat, they have also been advocating locally for improved dementia care and support.

Riversiders wanted to explore the experiences of people with dementia in relation to the GP annual review process. Annual reviews are specified in the General Practice Contract and reflected in their electronic record system. Group members felt that annual reviews were varied, with many people not having one. The group wanted to find out: (a) the proportion of people with dementia who had had an annual review at their GP practice; (b) the content and quality of the reviews;

and (c) whether the reviews were felt to be worthwhile by the person with dementia.

The group created a questionnaire – an online version and a paper copy – and circulated it through the DEEP (Dementia Engagement and Empowerment Project) network. Seventy-three questionnaires were completed. The results showed that few people with dementia get an annual review from their GP practice that is in any way meaningful to them, in terms of wellbeing and future planning. Care plans were only given to two people, and future care planning was not discussed at all (even though it is specified in the record system used by many GPs).

The group are aiming to engage with GPs and NHS England to improve annual reviews and primary care for people with dementia generally. To read the full report visit https://dementiaenquirers. org.uk/wp-content/uploads/2022/04/riversiders_annual-dementia-reviews_report-1.pdf.

Riversiders (Shrewsbury) with Minds and Voices (York): DEEP groups and Admiral Nurses working together

Riversiders and Minds and Voices were interested to know how much Admiral Nurses and DEEP (Dementia Engagement and Empowerment Project) groups interacted, if at all. They wanted to find out (a) how many Admiral Nurses knew about and met DEEP groups and (b) how many DEEP group members knew of and had access to Admiral Nurses. They created two different surveys, one for DEEP groups and one for Admiral Nurses.

They found that most Admiral Nurses had heard about DEEP, but not all were sure what DEEP was. Most thought it would be beneficial to have contact with a DEEP group, but only eight per cent had. Half of people with dementia had heard of Admiral Nurses, though only 17 per cent knew what Admiral Nurses did. Admiral Nurses and people with dementia could each see the benefits of making contact. Admiral Nurses saw the benefit in learning directly from people living with dementia; and people with dementia could see the benefits of Admiral Nurses providing support, knowledge and information.

Riversiders and Minds and Voices recommended that Admiral Nurses and DEEP groups explore opportunities to build relationships with each other. The project concluded with a fruitful meeting with Dementia

UK (which hosts Admiral Nurses) to implement the recommendations from the research project.

To read the full report visit https://dementiaenquirers.org.uk/ wp-content/uploads/2021/05/riversiders-in-shrewsbury-with-minds-and-voices-york_report.pdf.

Scottish Dementia Alumni (Scotland): Dementia Through Our Eyes resource

Scottish Dementia Alumni is a group of people living with different diagnoses of dementia for several years. They campaign with the wisdom of lived experience.

The group wanted to develop an interactive game for children aged between eight and ten to educate them about dementia. Raising awareness among children is a priority for Scottish Dementia Alumni 'so that everybody grows up knowing about dementia' (James McKillop). The group worked with Science Ceilidh in order to overcome group concerns about how challenging it might be to work in schools.

The project started with a framework for the game from Agnes, a group member. Children would move forward in steps for 'yes' or 'no' answers, with printable stepping stones, reaching a 'home' point. Game questions were developed by talking about what they needed children to know and their expertise. The game was tested out, by the group, with children in schools.

They noticed that the children changed their behaviour during the course of the game, as they learned about dementia. At first, they ran quickly to the answer points, not taking much time to think. But as the game progressed, they took much more time to re-read the possible answers and discuss between themselves which answer was best.

The group intend to develop the game further. The game and accompanying resources are available at www.scienceceilidh.com/ dementia-through-our-eyes?rq=dementia. To read the full report visit www.dementiavoices.org.uk/wp-content/uploads/2022/09/Scottish-Dementia-Alumni---August-2022.pdf.

SHINDIG (Sheffield): To drive or not to drive with dementia? That is the question

SHINDIG was formed in 2012 and is a forum where people living with dementia are supported to share their views, opinions and experiences of living with dementia in Sheffield.

SHINDIG wanted to explore the experience of driving, or having to stop driving, of people with dementia. This was an issue that was regularly discussed informally and at organized forums at SHINDIG meetings. The group felt that there should be a strong emphasis on safety and moral codes. They therefore applied successfully for formal ethical approval from a local university. Online interviews and focus groups were carried out.

The results of this project have not yet been made public as they are being written up for a dementia research journal. To read the full report visit https://dementiaenquirers.org.uk/wp-content/uploads/2022/08/dementia-enquirers-shindig-driving-report.pdf.

STAND (Fife): Contributing to the new Fife Dementia Strategy

STAND abbreviates Striving Towards A New Day. It is a peer support group for people with dementia and their family and friends. STAND also hosts a number of meeting centres.

STAND's project was one of five projects funded in response to the Covid-19 pandemic. This funding stream acknowledged the restrictions that would impact the way that projects could be delivered. The Fife Dementia Strategy was being refreshed at the time of this project. STAND members wanted to consult with people with dementia about what should go into the Dementia Strategy. They wanted to consult with people face-to-face with a blank sheet of paper and not on a formed strategy.

Sadly, Covid-19 had a major impact on the group's plans for this project. A questionnaire was developed by the Health and Social Care Partnership, and workshops were planned. However, uptake by people with dementia was low.

Subsequently, STAND were able to organize their own event in June 2022, as part of DEEP's (Dementia Engagement and Empowerment Project's) ten-year anniversary celebrations. Fifty people affected by dementia were in attendance. A blank sheet was given to people asking: 'What matters to you about living with dementia in Fife?' However, people found such an open-ended question to be too difficult. The priorities of STAND members were therefore used to guide discussions about what should be in the Fife Dementia Strategy:

- accessing self-directed support at an early stage in the disease process
- accessing peer support
- receiving care at home
- being actively involved in creative and artistic opportunities.

STAND learned a lot about running an enabling consultation with people with dementia. They are awaiting the report of their event, which will be fed into the Fife Dementia Strategy. To read the full report visit https://dementiaenquirers.org.uk/wp-content/uploads/2022/09/stand-in-fife.pdf.

SUNShiners (Dover, Deal and Shepway): Dementia as an invisible disability

SUNShiners is an activist group for people in the early stages of dementia; they aim to reduce stigma and raise public awareness. They also support the NHS through guiding recruitment and service development.

SUNShiners wanted to explore the invisibility of dementia, and the pros and cons of letting others know about their diagnoses. They were interested to find out: (a) what the public knew about dementia, (b) what they thought about the invisibility of dementia, and (c) why they might want to know if people have dementia.

The group created a questionnaire – an online version and a paper copy. Some of the questions were closed, and others were open-ended. The online version was circulated via friends and colleagues. The paper version was left in shops, cafes and groups, with a stamped addressed envelope.

The group were astounded to receive 347 responses to their survey! An academic researcher helped the group to think about the best ways to sort out these results and to make categories. The majority of people filling in the survey thought it was a negative that you can't always see dementia, because then others won't recognize symptoms and understand the experience. Most people thought that people with dementia should retain the right to vote and also that it would be helpful to know if someone had dementia on initial meeting.

People recognized that the answers were dependent on variabilities such as symptoms and access to support. To read the full report visit https://dementiaenquirers.org.uk/wp-content/uploads/2022/11/sunshiners-nov-2022.pdf.

Switchboard: The Space Between: Understanding the experiences of non-binary individuals with dementia

This research project was led by non-binary people with dementia, with the support of research allies in the field of dementia studies. Its objective was to explore the experiences of non-binary individuals with dementia and to identify the unique challenges they may face related to their gender identity.

This project used a qualitative approach to data collection and analysis, with semi-structured interviews. Participants were recruited through community organizations that support non-binary individuals, as well as through dementia support groups and healthcare providers.

The findings will be used to inform the development of more inclusive and culturally competent dementia care practices that take into account the diverse experiences of individuals with dementia.

THRED (Liverpool) Projects 1 and 2: Transport and dementia

The THRED group in Liverpool focus on improving local, regional and national transport systems to make them accessible and inclusive for people with dementia and their carers. Their strapline is 'Dementia, no barriers, no borders.'

THRED led a project to discover how urban and rural transport systems can help people diagnosed with dementia live independently for longer. They also had additional funding for a second project in response to the Covid-19 pandemic.

From their previous work, THRED knew that transport plays a major part in the quality of life of people with dementia and their carers. They decided to compare how people's experiences in rural areas differed from those in urban areas, and were interested to find out whether transport could promote independence or if it contributed to social isolation.

THRED met with people with dementia in England, Scotland and Northern Ireland, and held Zoom meetings with groups in North and Mid-Wales. They also created a survey that was completed by 57 people. From this research, they found that the majority of people with dementia were reliant on public transport. They regarded public transport as critical in staying connected. Helpful staff, accurate signage and information, and improved reliability of services would help people to use public transport more. There was a sense that transport providers did not do enough to encourage people with dementia (and other hidden disabilities) to feel confident to travel.

THRED concluded that public transport is important for people with dementia – it allows people to connect with places, and shapes how people live their lives. Increasing the support and awareness of dementia from public transport providers would benefit society and the economy and would also help people with dementia to feel more confident.

To read the full report visit https://dementiaenquirers.org.uk/wp-content/uploads/2021/05/thred-in-liverpool_report.pdf.

THRED (Liverpool) Project 3: Route to independence

THRED built on their previous Dementia Enquirers projects to explore what would help people with dementia build their confidence to travel by public transport.

They created a survey for people with dementia and carers. They also carried out some interviews. Additionally, they led discussions with train, bus and airport organizations to gather information. They asked people about their experiences of travelling by public transport, what would encourage people to use it more, and what plans they put in place to prepare for a journey.

THRED found that the biggest problems people with dementia experience when travelling by public transport were unhelpful staff and navigating transport hubs. Sixty per cent of people found travelling by public transport difficult. The most important areas to improve were availability, accessibility and signage.

From their findings, THRED has created a travel checklist for using public transport. They also recommend that transport providers read the report and address the barriers highlighted. To read the full report visit https://dementiaenquirers.org.uk/wp-content/uploads/2023/02/thred-route-to-independence-report.pdf.

Up and Go (Leeds): Can a dementia diagnosis open doors to new opportunities?

Up and Go is a group of people with dementia and supporters. They offer ideas that help their local community and environment to become more dementia friendly. They have a say in how local services are run and suggest how to improve them based on their experience and understanding of life with dementia.

Up and Go wanted to learn about how people with dementia in Yorkshire were taking up new opportunities. People with dementia in Up and Go have said that the group has opened up opportunities for them. They wanted to make sure other people with dementia were not missing out.

The group developed a survey to gather the opinions of people with dementia on the new opportunities they had, or did not have, following diagnosis. They also wanted to find out how people felt about this. The survey was online and in paper form. The group also had a field trip – to a llama farm! They reflected together afterwards on the impact of this new opportunity.

Of the people who filled in the survey, five in six had found a new opportunity after dementia diagnosis; two in three identified their new opportunity as starting a new group or activity; and one in six didn't have access to any new opportunities. The most common reasons for this were needing support to attend, or either not being bothered or lacking energy. The field trip showed that, with the right support in place, people with dementia can actively take up new opportunities that are enjoyable and socially-bonding experiences.

The group recommended, among other things, that new opportunities should be a priority after a dementia diagnosis. Professionals play a key role in helping newly diagnosed people to access groups and activities.

To read the full report visit https://dementiaenquirers.org.uk/wp-content/uploads/2022/11/up-and-go-leeds-oct-2022-report.pdf.

Case Studies

Case study 1: SUNShiners in Kent

The SUNShiners group ended up with a very large data set! They wanted to investigate what the general public know about dementia, what they thought about the invisibility of dementia, and why they might want to know if people have dementia. The group created a questionnaire and shared 100 print copies in shops, cafes and groups and also a SurveyMonkey online link.

They were delighted to receive 347 responses – and then completely overwhelmed! Especially as many of the questions were open-ended so people could write about their experiences in different ways – and at length!

So the group asked for help to analyse the data from a dementia researcher, Dr Rosie Ashworth. Rosie is experienced in co-research with people with dementia, is an advisor to the Dementia Enquirers programme, and was committed to making sure that people with dementia stayed 'in the driving seat' of this research. She supported SUNShiners to provide the parameters for the leg work that she was to carry out *on their behalf.*

This is what happened:

- SUNShiners thought about what reasons people may give for their answers.
- These formed the categories for Rosie to start sorting answers into.
- When Rosie had gone through several responses, she added

in categories that had come up, explaining to the SUNShiners why the data suggested these new categories.

- A set of criteria for what was put in each category was then given back to SUNShiners so that they could go through some more answers.
- Finally, Rosie grouped the rest of the answers following the same criteria.

The group were still in the driving seat of their research. As one SUNShiner said:

> It was important to get involved in a research project for a few reasons: to have a voice and to prove to people that we can still do things. Just because we have dementia doesn't mean we are unable to get involved. Our brains still work to a degree, just in a different way. I have enjoyed being part of the project and working as part of a team.

Case study 2: EDUCATE in Stockport

EDUCATE's report goes into very useful detail about the roles of the different project team members, and its authors are honest about some of the tensions that arose from a mismatch of expectations about what being 'in the driving seat' really means:

> Jacqui saw the Dementia Enquirers article in the DEEP [Dementia Engagement and Empowerment Project] newsletter and was inspired to take part with EDUCATE. She gave the printed synopsis of the grant to Ruth Chaplin, her keyworker, when she was visiting her house. In the application, Jacqui was put down as the lead of the project. Jacqui's understanding was that being 'in the driving seat' would mean that the project team (the people with dementia) would be in control of the project and make the decisions...not the professionals. However, Jacqui says: But this never happened. The professionals took charge of the project, which caused frustration and disappointment, as I felt that it should have been led and run by the project team. I was also disappointed that the project team members could not, due to General Data Protection Regulation,

accompany Rebecca on the installation and follow-up visits. In the event, Jacqui took on the role of writing up/editing the report, using the information given by Rebecca and Mark, and input from the project team.

In 2015, Steve Clifford had been involved in an EU robotics project, testing a domiciliary 'care bot'. At the time, he questioned the value of spending millions on a robot when a lot of its functions could be carried out by Alexa. Steve's insight created the momentum leading to this enquiry. Steve feels that: 'We've steered it in the way we wanted it to go... The information we produced is very good, it's very clear.'

Joan Palmer has embraced the challenge of technology throughout the ten years she has lived with dementia, often describing the frustration and anxiety she experienced when things don't work. Joan was also involved in a Super Mario (digital game) project, helping test functionality and identifying barriers to use. She brought home to us the importance of relational support in overcoming barriers to using technology, by describing how her grandson was able to explain things to her in a way others couldn't. When asked if she had been given an opportunity to be in the driving seat of the project, Joan said: We all go around and we say how we've been using it [Alexa]. I speak up; that's being in the driving seat isn't it? [But] sometimes it goes over my head when we're talking about it. If I had to do anything like writing or designing logos, I'd be up all night worrying about it. One or two of the others could do that – they'd be well away! I think we've covered everything; it's been really good. I'm looking forward to reading the final report.

Joan gave a presentation about the project to the Pennine Care NHS Foundation Trust's Occupational Therapy Conference in November 2019. She found sharing her story at the conference very affirming, and her presentation featured in the monthly blog of Pennine Care's CEO Claire Molloy, who wrote: I loved hearing about their (virtual personal assistant) Alexa project, which is changing some of our service users' lives in remarkable ways. This work is helping people stay independent, with Alexa reminding them to take medication, attend appointments and do exercises, as well as assisting them to order food and taxis, dictate texts and get help.

Alan Bancroft was away in the USA for part of the project, but when involved, he was an active and insightful participant. His view is that: I don't think any one person can be 'in the driving seat': it's more like we all were. So you'll need a minivan! I would need more one-to-one, face-to-face support to go through the report, line by line, as it were. Unfortunately, that's not possible at the moment (due to Coronavirus). Overall, the important thing has been about finding out how it can help people with dementia and other illnesses. In my case, that would be help with my language. I was interested to see that someone testing Alexa had help with something called 'errorless learning techniques'. I now want to know if that could help me, not just with Alexa, but generally.

Caron Anderton played a very valuable role, offering many concrete suggestions. When asked about being in the driving seat, she says: I've been able to learn from the others at the meetings, because they know more about this than I do. I get panicky if I get too much information at once, because it's too much to take in... So it's been about learning. It's been really good for me.

Finally, Mark Perry, one of the facilitators, comments: We've approached the enquiry as a partnership. Our questions to the project team as facilitators were: 'What can you as people with dementia teach us about Alexa that can help others using or designing this kind of technology? You've asked some questions about Alexa; how can we help you answer them?' We've tried to help by providing sufficient occupational therapy input to allow people with dementia the time and space to discuss, set up and practise using Alexa. This has enabled participants to explain its uses, benefits and problems to us in their own personal and environmental context. We have been inclusive, bringing together people living with a range of diagnoses, abilities and problems, enabling the testing of Alexa in unique personal circumstances. The explanations provided by the participants have been shared with project team members, who have also contributed their own, and been used to help answer the project team's original questions.

While facilitators have made opportunities available to people with dementia to take on project team work – chairing meetings, designing logos, helping design feedback forms and writing the report – most project team members were clear they did not want these roles and identified some of them as overwhelming. By answering their questions, project members wanted to learn about Alexa and help others to do the same. They did this as experts by experience, using their ability to learn and teach at the same time, helping to produce the valuable information that can now be shared and evaluated. This approach comes naturally to group members, as they have been using it for many years when helping deliver dementia training. This is our take on 'being in the driving seat'.

In conclusion, this project has very usefully highlighted the ambiguity of the 'driving seat' aspiration, and the many different ways in which it can be interpreted. One member felt that she could and should be in a real leadership role (with assistance where needed), while other team members, and the group facilitators, felt that the main fieldwork and data collection should be done by a professional, with the project team as advisors. This misunderstanding led to some changes in the support arrangements mid-project. It is fair to say that this caused a certain amount of difficulty for the project – which, with hindsight, could have been reduced by very early agreement about expectations, skillsets and roles. However, this is valuable learning for both Dementia Enquirers and EDUCATE.

Conference and Seminar Presentations

2019

- UK Dementia Congress

2020

- Dementia Action Alliance Webinar
- Dementia Care UK Research Summit (National Institute of Health and Care Research, Economic and Social Research Council, Alzheimer's Society)
- Seminar for London School of Hygiene and Tropical Medicine
- Podcast by the Pioneers as part of National Co-Production Week
- British Society of Gerontology Annual Conference
- Presentation to the University of Bradford

2021

- NIHR (National Institute for Health and Care Research) Webinar
- NHS Tayside – Dementia Research Summit
- Research in Practice for Adults webinar
- Seminar on Public Involvement for NIHR Research Design Service, Yorkshire and Humber

- Presentation to the University of West London Young Dementia Network

2022

- Alzheimer's Disease International Conference
- UK Dementia Congress
- Masterclass for Early Career Researchers
- Masterclass for the University of Stirling School of Dementia Studies
- Alzheimer's Europe Conference
- Research in Practice Leaders' Forum

2023

- UK Dementia Congress
- Alzheimer's Europe Conference

References

Barnes, C. (2001) '"Emancipatory" Disability Research: Project or Process?' Public Lecture at City Chambers, Glasgow.

Berry, P., Davies, T., Fordyce, C., Gordon, H., Houston, A. *et al.* (2019) 'Dementia Enquirers – People with dementia in the driving seat of research.' *Dementia*, 19(1), 68–73.

British Psychological Society (2021) *BPS Code of Human Research Ethics*. Available at: www.bps.org.uk/guideline/bps-code-human-research-ethics.

British Society of Gerontology (2012) BSG Ethical Guidelines. Available at: www. britishgerontology.org/about-bsg/bsg-ethical-guidelines.

Buffel, T. & James, H. (2019) 'Working with older people as co-researchers in developing age friendly communities.' *Gerontology*, 21(2).

Clough, R., Green, B., Hawkes, B., Raymond, G. & Bright, L. (2006) *Older People as Researchers: Evaluating a Participative Project*. London: Joseph Rowntree Foundation.

Davies, T., Houston, A., Gordon, H., McLintock, M., *et al.* (2021) 'Dementia Enquirers: Pioneering approaches to dementia research in the UK.' *Disability and Society*, 37(1), 129–147.

Economic and Social Research Council (2022) *Framework for Research Ethics*. Available at: https://www.ukri.org/councils/esrc/guidance-for-applicants/research-ethics-guidance/framework-for-research-ethics/

Faulkner, A. & Layzell, S. (2000) *Strategies for Living: A Report of User Led Research into People's Strategies for Living with Mental Distress*. London: Mental Health Foundation.

Fricker, M. (2007) *Epistemic Injustice: Power & the Ethics of Knowing*. Oxford: Oxford University Press.

Health Research Authority (HRA) *Health Research Authority Decision Tools*. Available at: https://www.hra-decisiontools.org.uk/research/

Houston, A. (2017) *Dementia and Sensory Challenges: Dementia can be More Than Memory*. Glasgow: Life Changes Trust.

Innovations in Dementia (2017) *Our Lived Experience: Current Evidence on Dementia Rights in the UK*. An alternative report to the UN CRPD committee. Exeter: Innovations in Dementia.

Innovations in Dementia (2020) *The Right to a Grand Day Out: A Story of Co-Production.* Exeter: Innovations in Dementia.

Innovations in Dementia (2021) *My Life, My Goals.* Exeter: Innovations in Dementia. Available at: www.innovationsindementia.org.uk/2021/09/my-life-my-goals.

Innovations in Dementia (2022) *Top Tips for Facilitators: Ideas from a DEEP Facilitators' Gathering.* Exeter: Innovations in Dementia.

Innovations in Dementia (2023a) *How To Do a Research Project.* Exeter: Innovations in Dementia.

Innovations in Dementia (2023b) *The Dementia Enquirers Gold Standards for Ethical Research.* Exeter: Innovations in Dementia.

Innovations in Dementia (2023c) *How to Write and Produce Better Information for People with Dementia.* Exeter: Innovations in Dementia.

James, H. & Buffel, T. (2022) 'Co-research with older people: A systematic literature review.' *Ageing and Society*, 1–27. doi:10.1017/S0144686X21002014.

Liabo, K., Cockcroft, E., Boddy, K., Farmer, L., Bortoli, S. & Britten, N. (2022) 'Epistemic justice in public involvement and engagement: Creating conditions for impact.' *Health Expectations*, 25(4), 1967–1978.

Litherland, R. (2015) *Developing a National User Movement of People with Dementia.* Joseph Rowntree Foundation. Available at: www.jrf.org.uk/report/developing-national-user-movement-people-dementia.

Mayer, J.D. & Gaschke, Y.N. (1988) 'The experience and meta-experience of mood.' *Journal of Personality and Social Psychology*, 55, 102–111.

National Institute for Health and Care Research (2021) *Briefing Note 3: Why Involve Members of the Public in Research?* Available at: www.nihr.ac.uk/documents/briefing-notes-for-researchers-public-involvement-in-nhs-health-and-social-care-research/27371#briefing-note-three-why-involve-members-of-the-public-in-research.

New Economics Foundation (2008) *Co-production: A Manifesto for Growing the Core Economy.* London: NEF.

NHS Health Research Authority (n.d.) *Research Ethics Service and Research Ethics Committees.* Available at: www.hra.nhs.uk/about-us/committees-and-services/res-and-recs.

Oliver, M. (1992) 'Changing the social relations of research production?' *Disability, Handicap & Society*, 7(2), 101–114, doi: 10.1080/02674649266780141.

Scottish Dementia Working Group, Research Sub-group (2013) *Core Principles for Involving People with Dementia in Research.* Available at: http://dementiavoices.org.uk/wp-content/uploads/2014/06/Involving-people-with-dementia-in-research1.pdf.

Staley, K. (2009) *Exploring Impact: Public Involvement in NHS, Public Health and Social Care Research.* Eastleigh: INVOLVE.

Tuffrey-Wijne, I., Kar Kei Lam, C., Marsden, B., Harris, C. *et al.* (2020) 'Developing a training course to teach research skills to people with learning disabilities: "It gives us a voice. We CAN be researchers!"' *British Journal of Learning Disabilities*, 48(4), 301–314.

UK Research and Innovation (n.d.) *Research Ethics Guidance*. Available at: www.ukri.org/councils/esrc/guidance-for-applicants/research-ethics-guidance.

Wallcraft, J. & Sweeney, A. (2003) *On Our Own Terms: Users and Survivors of Mental Health Services Working Together for Support and Change*. London: Sainsbury Centre for Mental Health.

Wellcome Trust (2014) *Ensuring Your Research is Ethical: A Guide for Extended Project Qualification Students*. Available at: https://wellcome.org/sites/default/files/wtp057673_0.pdf.

Wilkinson, H. (2001) *The Perspectives of People with Dementia: Research Methods and Motivations*. London and Philadelphia: Jessica Kingsley Publishers.

World Health Organization (2017) *Global Action Plan on the Public Health Response to Dementia 2017–2025*. Geneva: WHO.